LETTING GO OF
PERFECT

LETTING GO OF
PERFECT

Overcoming Perfectionism in Kids

JILL L. ADELSON, PH.D.,
and HOPE E. WILSON, PH.D.

PRUFROCK PRESS INC.
WACO, TEXAS

Library of Congress Cataloging-in-Publication Data

Adelson, Jill L., 1979-
  Letting go of perfect : overcoming perfectionism in kids / Jill L. Adelson and Hope E. Wilson.
    p. cm.
  Includes bibliographical references.
  ISBN-13: 978-1-59363-362-2 (pbk.)
  ISBN-10: 1-59363-362-9 (pbk.)
  1. Perfectionism (Personality trait) 2. Children. I. Wilson, Hope E., 1980- II. Title.
  BF698.35.P47A34 2009
  155.4'18232--dc22
                            2009005801

Edited by Lacy Compton
Cover and Layout Design by Marjorie Parker
Illustrated by David Parker

ISBN-13: 978-1-59363-362-2
ISBN-10: 1-59363-362-9

Printed in the United States of America.

At the time of this book's publication, all facts and figures cited are the most current available. All telephone numbers, addresses, and Web site URLs are accurate and active. All publications, organizations, Web sites, and other resources exist as described in the book, and all have been verified. The authors and Prufrock Press Inc., make no warranty or guarantee concerning the information and materials given out by organizations or content found at Web sites, and we are not responsible for any changes that occur after this book's publication. If you find an error, please contact Prufrock Press Inc.

Prufrock Press Inc.
P.O. Box 8813
Waco, TX 76714-8813
Phone: (800) 998-2208
Fax: (800) 240-0333
http://www.prufrock.com

DEDICATION

This book is dedicated to my husband, Jon, whose patience, belief in me, and support has helped me use my own perfectionism to accomplish many things, including the writing of this book. It also is dedicated to my former students at B. C. Charles who taught me at least as much as I taught them.—Jill

This book is dedicated to my supportive husband, Jon, and my children, Lily and Keenan, who have supported me throughout this journey.—Hope

CONTENTS

ACKNOWLEDGMENTS

WE both would like to acknowledge and thank those who inspired us to study perfectionism. Hope was inspired by the work and research of her friend, Pat Schuler; and Jill was inspired and encouraged by her friend (and then professor at The College of William and Mary), Catherine Little, and the outstanding young students in her fourth-grade class. We also would like to acknowledge the help and valuable advice from our advisors and friends at the University of Connecticut, including Kathy Gavin, Jean Gubbins, Catherine Little, Betsy McCoach, Sally Reis, Joe Renzulli, and Del Siegle.

This book would not be possible without Lacy Compton of Prufrock Press. We owe her many thanks for recognizing the potential for this book, for providing invaluable suggestions to improve it, and for supporting us, especially in our moments of being Procrastinating Perfectionists.

We also would like to thank Mrs. Nancy Titchen for trying some of our suggestions with her students.

1

PERFECTIONISM AND CHILDREN

CHANCES are that you are reading this book because you are concerned about a child, either your own or one in your class, who has exhibited **perfectionistic behaviors**. It may be that you are concerned about the child's stress levels, the lack of joy the child takes in the process of creating, or the overly developed **self-criticism** he or she demonstrates. Perhaps your child has an obsession with mistakes and "flaws," sheds tears over small errors and perceived imperfections, or tends toward **procrastination** and **fear of failure**. When perfectionism becomes unhealthy, we, as adults, become concerned for our children and want to help them, but we often are at a loss for what to do.

In the roles of parent and teacher, we have struggled with how to help children use their **perfectionism** in a healthy way instead of becoming paralyzed, frustrated, anxious, and stressed. This book stemmed from a case study observing Jill's fourth graders and noting their perfectionistic behaviors (Adelson, 2007). From this case study, she identified five types of perfectionism. Between the two of us, we have worked with hundreds of children, including Hope's own child, and have had the opportunity to use the strategies we suggest. Of course, there is no one solution to helping your child use his or her perfectionism in a healthy way. Hopefully,

Note that words in **bold** are defined in the glossary in the back of the book!

this book will give you some ideas that will help you work with your child and create an environment that encourages risk-taking, acknowledges mistakes as learning experiences, supports short-term as well as long-term goal setting, and celebrates accomplishments, the process, and personal areas of strength. As a parent and/or teacher, you can serve as a role model, support system, and a source of guidance to a child with perfectionism. With your help, your child can let go of unhealthy perfectionism. However, it will not happen overnight. This process takes time. As Corinne, one of Jill's former fourth-grade students, said, "Really, the only way to overcome perfectionism is to accept it and consistently tell yourself it doesn't have to be perfect. Over time, with the maturity of growing up and the consistency of your corrections, it will level out." To help the children we love, we must help them both to understand their perfectionistic tendencies and to learn to use their perfectionism in healthy ways.

> "Really, the only way to overcome perfectionism is to accept it and consistently tell yourself it doesn't have to be perfect. . . ."
> —Corinne, Newport News, VA

If your child talks about suicide, seems depressed, or stops eating, be sure to seek professional help. The strategies in this book are meant as a guide for parents and teachers to help children who are struggling with unhealthy perfectionism. However, perfectionism can lead to more serious conditions, such as **suicide, eating disorders, depression**, and **anxiety disorders**. There are many resources concerning anxiety in children available to parents. Some of these are included in Chapters 11 and 12, which provide resources for parents and children. Perfectionism also can be a symptom of many of these underlying psychological issues. If you feel that your child, at any point, may be experiencing more serious signs of psychological distress, please seek the professional help of a licensed psychologist, psychiatrist, counselor, or therapist. Signs for concern might include a change in mood, loss of appetite, change in eating habits, depression, talk of death or suicide, change in personality, or change in sleeping patterns.

HEALTHY AND UNHEALTHY PERFECTIONISM

No one is a perfectionist in all parts of his or her life at all times. In general, we tend to refer to perfectionistic behaviors or **perfectionistic tendencies** rather than to perfectionists, recognizing that perfectionism can be exhibited under various circumstances throughout a person's life. Your decision to read this book suggests that you have recognized perfectionistic behaviors in a child you want to help. What many people do not realize is that perfectionism can be used in both healthy and unhealthy ways, often referred to as **adaptive perfectionism** and **maladaptive perfectionism**. Instead, people often only refer to someone as a perfectionist in a negative way. They focus on the stress, anxiety, fear, and procrastination that can result from perfectionistic behaviors. However, when used in a healthy way, perfectionism can result in a focus on improvement through revision and practice, in goal setting, and in motivation to develop one's potential and abilities.

Your child might exhibit characteristics of more than one of the five types of perfectionists that we describe.

According to Hamachek (1978), who used the term "**normal**" to refer to healthy perfectionism and the term "**neurotic**" to refer to unhealthy perfectionism, children who use their perfectionism in healthy ways "derive a real sense of pleasure from the labors of a painstaking effort" and they "feel free to be less precise as the situation permits" (p. 27). This is the goal we want for children exhibiting perfectionism. We hope the strategies suggested in this book will help you move children toward this type of orientation, taking pleasure in the process and recognizing that they do not need to strive for perfection at all times.

ABOUT THIS BOOK

The next chapter of this book provides you more background information about perfectionism. We provide you an overview of the research on perfectionism by debunking seven myths about perfectionism. This chapter will help you understand some common misconceptions about perfectionism and how these myths might apply to your child.

Chapters 3 through 7 introduce each of the five types of perfectionists identified in the article "A 'Perfect' Case Study: Perfectionism in Academically Talented Fourth Graders," published in *Gifted Child Today* (Adelson, 2007). The five types are the **Academic Achiever**, the **Aggravated Accuracy Assessor**, the **Risk Evader**, the **Controlling Image Manager**, and the **Procrastinating Perfectionist**. First, we present vignettes that describe children exhibiting behaviors characteristic of that type of perfectionist. These are based on the children we have worked with and have observed. Then, we describe the characteristics of that type of perfectionist. Following the description, we provide strategies for the classroom and for the home to help students who exhibit this type of perfectionism use it in a healthy manner.

After the five types of perfectionism, we help you identify healthy and unhealthy perfectionism. This chapter, Chapter 8, includes a list of behaviors characteristic of each of the five types of perfectionists, a list of signs of unhealthy perfectionism, a description of healthy perfectionists, and a list of tools you can use to identify perfectionistic tendencies in children.

Having established what perfectionism is, noting the differences between healthy and unhealthy perfections and examining the five types of perfectionism, we then provide what many teachers and parents are wanting—an overview of strategies to help children use perfectionism in a healthy way in the classroom (Chapter 9) and in the home (Chapter 10). Each of these chapters begins with a table reviewing the strategies we recommend for each of the five types of perfectionism. Although we encourage you to read the individual chapters for more detailed descriptions, this provides a summary of those strategies. In Chapter 9, we share general strategies for the classroom, which are followed by specific activities for the classroom. These include suggestions to be used within existing classroom activities like pretesting and posttesting, and they also include specific activities addressing perfectionism. In Chapter 10, we review the strategies for the five types of perfectionism with methods to be used in "**crisis moments**." Next, we provided general strategies and discussion suggestions for you and your child as well as suggestions for family time. This chapter ends by addressing a time during which many parents struggle to help their child with perfectionism—homework time.

Our goal is not to eliminate having high goals and standards but to help children take pleasure in the process, appreciate their strengths, see their mistakes as learning experiences, and recognize that they should not expect perfection at all times.

We hope you will find this book helpful for creating a positive environment and supporting your young child who is experiencing perfectionism. However, there are other resources to help you further. In Chapter 11, we provide some suggested resources for children, including books, Web sites, games, and programs. Then in Chapter 12, we provide resources for adults, including books, articles, Web sites, and organizations.

At the end of this book you will find a glossary and a list of references. We have provided definitions for each of the bold words in the book. The references are a good resource if you want to read more about research on perfectionism, especially in **gifted children**.

2

DEBUNKING MYTHS ABOUT PERFECTIONISM

MANY teachers and parents have misconceptions about perfectionism, especially in gifted children. This chapter will outline seven of the most common beliefs about perfectionism and what researchers have found to support or to debunk them. Researchers in this field have used **scientific** and **observational techniques** to learn about perfectionism among both adults and children. To give you an understanding of this research, we will share with you how it applies to commonly held beliefs about perfectionism. In addition, we will provide practical applications for each myth, showing how it applies to the children in your life. Table 1 provides the seven myths about perfectionism.

MYTH 1: PERFECTIONISM IS ALWAYS BAD FOR CHILDREN

Parents and teachers tend to talk about perfectionism as a negative trait among their children. The words, "That Julia, she is such a perfectionist. Why can't she just let go of those mistakes?" or "I just wish that I could stop Marcos from being such a perfectionist" often

TABLE 1

The Seven Myths About Perfectionism

1. Perfectionism is always bad for children.
2. Only gifted children are perfectionists.
3. No one knows why some children are perfectionists.
4. There are no ways to identify perfectionism.
5. Adults cannot do anything to help young perfectionists.
6. There is only one type of perfectionist.
7. Perfectionism is not really that harmful for children.

are heard in teachers' lounges and at parent meetings. Certainly, these parents and teachers never discuss the positive aspects of perfectionism. However, the children being discussed often are some of the highest achieving and motivated students in the class. So, perhaps there also are positive qualities to perfectionism.

What the Research Says

In fact, researchers emphasize two aspects of perfectionism: healthy and unhealthy. Basically, the characteristics of perfectionism either can enhance a child's achievement and well-being or can be damaging to self-esteem and success. **Healthy perfectionism**, sometimes called *normal* or *adaptive perfectionism*, represents the characteristics that are positive for students, including gaining a sense of pride from achievements and a drive for success. **Unhealthy perfectionism**, sometimes called *neurotic* or *maladaptive perfectionism*, is the type of perfectionism that most often comes to mind when parents and teachers think of their children. It represents the perfectionism that causes concern about a student's behavior and well-being. Table 2 provides a look at the differences between healthy and unhealthy perfectionism.

Table 2

Differences Between Healthy and Unhealthy Perfectionism

Healthy Perfectionism	Unhealthy Perfectionism
High, yet realistic standards	Unrealistic standards
Gains pleasure from working hard at difficult tasks	Often unsatisfied with high levels of effort
Capable of choosing to relax standards depending on task	Unable to relax standards
Motivation based on personal standards concerning work effort	Motivation based on external evaluations of product
Mastery-oriented	Performance-oriented
Conscientious	Low self-esteem

Note. From Blankstein, Dunkley, and Wilson (2008); Hamachek (1978); Stumpf and Parker (2000).

Other researchers classify these types of perfectionists in terms of their **motivation**. Healthy perfectionists seem to derive their motivation from personal standards for effort and work, while unhealthy perfectionists tend to base their motivation on evaluative concerns. Thus, healthy perfectionists may be more concerned with obtaining mastery of a given skill, while unhealthy perfectionists are more concerned with how they perform that skill.

Healthy perfectionism can enhance a child's achievement and well-being, but unhealthy perfectionism can damage a child's self-esteem and success.

In addition, some researchers classify healthy and unhealthy perfectionism as dichotomous characteristics, meaning that a student is one or the other (Hamachek, 1978; Hawkins, Watt, & Sinclair, 2006; Parker, 1997; Parker, Flett, & Hewitt, 2002). However, other researchers conceptualize these as two ends of a continuum in which most perfectionists lie somewhere in the middle (Schuler, 2000). The distinctions between healthy and unhealthy perfectionists have been seen in cultures around the world (Schuler et al., 2003).

Many researchers have found that students who are perfectionists have higher levels of achievement. In one study, college-aged perfectionists had higher grade point averages than their nonperfectionistic peers (Gilman & Ashby, 2003; Witcher, Alexander, Onwuebuzie, Collins, & Witcher, 2007). Another study also documented higher grade point averages among female students who were perfectionists than among their nonperfectionistic peers (Must, 2008).

Additionally, research suggests that healthy perfectionists have higher satisfaction with all aspects of their life than maladapative perfectionists, but both types of perfectionists have higher life satisfaction than nonperfectionists (Gilman & Ashby, 2003). In middle school, healthy perfectionists report having more positive peer relationships and lower levels of social stress than unhealthy perfectionists (Gilman & Ashby, 2003). Similar results were found for athletes (Immundsen, Roberts, Lemyre, & Miller, 2005). Finally, a study showed that among college students, healthy perfectionists have more pride and less shame and guilt than unhealthy perfectionists (Stoeber, Harris, & Moon, 2007).

Final Thoughts

Although most people think of perfectionism as a negative characteristic, research shows that perfectionism can be either healthy or unhealthy. When students use high personal standards and mastery-orientation to motivate themselves toward higher levels of success, it can lead to greater achievement, more positive social relationships, and greater life satisfaction. The key for parents and teachers is to encourage children to move from unhealthy to healthy types of perfectionism. Strategies for this will be provided in subsequent chapters.

MYTH 2: ONLY GIFTED CHILDREN ARE PERFECTIONISTS

Many parents, teachers, researchers, and authors have character-ized perfectionism as a problem that only affects the gifted population (Callard-Szulgit, 2003). Perfectionism is a condition that often is addressed in textbooks and materials con-cerning the social and emotional devel-opment of gifted students. Teachers tend to associate perfectionism primarily with students who they believe have high abilities or potential.

"The key for parents and teachers is to encourage children to move from unhealthy to healthy types of perfectionism."

What the Research Says

Research, on the other hand, does not support this opinion. Although many researchers and professionals in the field of gifted edu-cation conceptualize perfectionism as a problem primarily for gifted students, many studies have shown perfectionism among students of varying ability levels. For example, when giving perfectionism scales to students of all ability levels, studies show that students identified as gifted are no more likely to exhibit perfectionistic tendencies (Green-spon, 2008; Parker, 2000; Parker & Mills, 1996). In fact, there is some evidence that students with higher levels of perfectionism score lower on **creativity tests**, a common indicator of giftedness among students (Gallucci, Middleton, & Kline, 2000). Other research indicates that gifted students actually have higher healthy perfectionism scores but lower unhealthy scores (LoCicero & Ashby, 2000), indicating that gifted students may be better able to handle higher standards without damaging self-esteem.

Other research indicates that students with varying levels of ability also experience perfectionism. In fact, many studies have shown the prevalence of perfectionism among samples that include subjects from diverse levels of ability (e.g., Flett, Hewitt, Blankenstein, & Pickering, 1998; Frost & Marten, 1990; Suddarth & Slaney, 2001). Studies of college students found perfectionism among students with learning disabilities (O'Brien, 2006; Saddler & Buckland, 1995). Perfectionism was found in populations of both above-average and average-ability mathematics students in the Czech Republic (Parker, Portesova, & Stumpf, 2001). Thus, it is apparent from research that perfectionism can affect students of varying ability levels.

Final Thoughts

Perfectionism certainly is an issue that is associated closely with gifted students, but that does not necessarily indicate that the gifted population is more likely to exhibit perfectionistic tendencies than the general population. Children may direct perfectionism toward varying aspects of their lives, such as athletics, fine arts, or hobbies. **Academically gifted children** may be more likely to direct their perfectionism toward schoolwork, thus capturing the attention of teachers and parents. It is important for teachers and parents of all children to be aware of the negative aspects of unhealthy perfectionism and to provide opportunities for students to adapt their characteristics to a more positive approach.

MYTH 3: NO ONE KNOWS WHY SOME CHILDREN ARE PERFECTIONISTS

Parents and teachers tend to throw up their hands in confusion as to why some children seem to exhibit perfectionistic tendencies more than others. Certainly, perfectionism is a product of a person's personality, but what factors contribute to it? Although there is no formula that results in perfectionism, researchers have shown that some characteristics of a child's environment can contribute.

What the Research Says

One personality factor that research has linked to perfectionism is **dichotomous thinking**. Dichotomous thinking is the tendency to view events in life as either bad or good, with little or no "gray area" in between. When tasks are seen as either complete successes or failures, and by association, the sense of self becomes either a success or failure, perfectionism is a natural consequence (Egan, Piek, Dyck, & Rees, 2007). Any error or mistake can lead a child with dichotomous thinking to believe that he or she is a complete failure.

The circumstances of a child's environment may contribute to perfectionism. Birth order is one example of an environmental factor in perfectionism. Some studies have shown that firstborn children are more likely to exhibit perfectionistic behaviors (Siegle & Schuler, 2000). Children of alcoholics also seem to be more prone to perfectionism (Gaspar, 2007).

Parents may influence their child's tendency toward perfectionism in a number of ways. For instance, a parent's own perfectionism may be a contributor to a child's perfectionism. In a study of college females, researchers found that their mother's perfectionism was more closely associated with their perfectionism than that of their father (Frost, Lahart, & Rosnblate, 1991). However, other research found no link between parental and child perfectionism (Dekryger, 2006). **Parenting style** also seems to have a factor in perfectionism. Harshness in parenting and use of control has been linked to higher levels of perfectionism in daughters (Frost et al., 1991; Kenney-Benson & Pomerantz, 2005). The group with the highest levels of perfectionism were firstborn children with high levels of parental criticism and expectations (Siegle & Schuler, 2000).

Other researchers have found that inconsistent or nonexistent approval from parents also can lead to perfectionism in children, as can parental approval that is conditional to a child's performance (Hamachek, 1978). A parent's ability to nurture children (Diprima, 2003) as well as his or her focus on **learning goals** rather than **performance goals** (Ablard & Parker, 1997) makes a difference in a child developing healthy or unhealthy perfectionism. American parents of perfectionists tend to have high standards for their children and have a high need for organization (O'Leary & Schuler, 2003). Finally, family environments that focus on high achievement, are punitive, and have structured environments have significantly higher levels of perfectionism than families with flexible and **task-involving environments** (McArdle & Duda, 2004). In this type of environment, parents are involved with their children in everyday tasks and family activities. Parenting style and family environment clearly impact the development of perfectionism in children.

A child's tendency toward perfectionism may be influenced by his or her parents.

Final Thoughts

Some factors contributing to perfectionism cannot be changed, such as birth order. However, other personality and environmental contributors can be altered to help children's perfectionism be used in healthy rather than unhealthy ways. Parents, teachers, and counselors can work with children to change dichotomous thinking into a healthier mode of perception, recognizing that mistakes are acceptable and that a flaw does not make a person a failure. Parenting styles that focus on mistakes, performance goals, and harshness and that withhold acceptance may contribute to perfectionism among children. Adapting a parenting style that focuses more on learning from mistakes and on positive accomplishments in all tasks may help children develop healthy, rather than unhealthy, perfectionism.

MYTH 4: THERE ARE NO WAYS TO IDENTIFY PERFECTIONISM

Parents and teachers often wonder if there is a formal way to identify the children in their lives who might be perfectionists. Aside from the vast amount of anecdotal information that parents and teachers gather every day about a child's behavior, attitudes, and thought processes, adults would like a uniform way to measure the perfectionism in children. Fortunately, researchers have developed a variety of measures of perfectionism. In addition, specialists in the field have identified common characteristics of students who are perfectionists.

What the Research Says

The **instruments** available to measure perfectionism reflect the theories held by the authors and developers of each test. The Conners' Parent Rating Scale (Conners, Sitarenios, Parker, & Epstein, 1998a) and the Conners' Teacher Rating Scale (Conners, Sitarenios, Parker, & Epstein, 1998b) measure what the authors consider factors of perfectionism, including being fussy, doing things the same way, getting upset if things move, being overfocused, and neatness. The Multidimensional Perfectionism Scale (Parker & Stumpf, 1995; Sondergeld, Schultz, & Glover, 2007) measures both unhealthy and healthy perfectionism in students, and it has been expanded to the Childhood Multidimensional Perfectionism Scale (Dekryger, 2006). Other measures include the Child and Adolescent Perfectionism Scale (Castro et al., 2004; McCreary, Joiner, Schmidt, & Ialongo, 2004), the

Almost Perfect Scale-Revised (Rice, Ashby, & Slaney, 2007; Vandiver & Worrell, 2002), the Adaptive/Maladaptive Perfectionism Scale (Rice & Dellwo, 2002; Rice, Kubal, & Preusser, 2004; Rice, Leever, Noggle, & Lapsley, 2007), and the Perfectionism Cognitions Inventory (Flett, Hewitt, Whelan, & Martin, 2007). These instruments have been used in both research and clinical settings.

Sometimes a measure of perfectionism is part of a larger instrument, such as the Smith Irrational Beliefs Inventory (Amutio & Smith, 2007; Smith, Rausch, & Jenks, 2004), the Student Adjustment Problems Inventory (Chan, 2003), and the Multidimensional Anxiety Scale for Children (MASC; March, Parker, Sullivan, & Stallings, 1997). These tend to measure unhealthy forms of perfectionism and view perfectionism as a contributing factor toward anxiety or other forms of psychological distress.

Many perfectionists focus on mistakes and the consequences of those mistakes.

These types of instruments are used by researchers and professionals to diagnose perfectionism. They are designed to be used by people who are trained in assessment procedures and familiar with research methodologies. Parents are advised against using these instruments with their own children. Instead, interested parents and family members can contact professional psychologists or school personnel to administer assessments to diagnose perfectionism.

In addition to the formal instruments that have been developed to measure perfectionism in children, researchers also have developed lists of characteristics of perfectionism. Lists of characteristics can be helpful for parents and teachers to identify children who may be in need of additional support. These characteristics include fear of failure, dichotomous thinking, procrastination, low **self-esteem** based on external rewards, underachievement, and a tendency to overwork (Adderholdt-Elliot, 1989). Researchers studying children identified as demonstrating perfectionistic behaviors observed them in play

Table 3

Characteristics of Unhealthy Perfectionists From Research

1.	Fear of failure
2.	Procrastination
3.	Dichotomous thinking
4.	Low self-esteem
5.	Concentration on external rewards
6.	Workaholic tendencies
7.	Underachievement
8.	Focus on mistakes
9.	Greater levels of anxiety
10.	Minor mistakes generalized to overall low self-esteem

Note. From Adderholdt-Elliot (1989); and Ashby et al. (2004).

settings. They found that often the themes of these children's play center around mistakes and consequences for mistakes or imperfections, rather than around living up to personal or external standards. These children have internalized their dichotomous thinking so that they generalize minor mistakes, resulting in low **self-concept**. Children demonstrating perfectionism also demonstrate greater levels of anxiety throughout their play sessions (Ashby, Kottman, & Martin, 2004). A summary of the research on the characteristics of unhealthy perfectionists can be found in Table 3.

Final Thoughts

Experts in the field of perfectionism have developed a wide variety of measures. These can be found throughout the journals articles and books that have been written about perfectionism that are listed in the reference section of this book. Less formal assessment can be made through the use of checklists that are mentioned in this and other chapters in this book. For instance, in Chapter 8, we include the following lists: behaviors typical of the five types of perfectionists we address in the book, the signs of unhealthy perfectionism, and skills for healthy perfectionism. All of these resources can be used to help identify students who may be in danger of developing unhealthy perfectionism. Again, the key is not to focus on identifying perfectionistic behaviors in hopes of eliminating them, but on identifying unhealthy manifestations of perfectionism and helping students use their perfectionism in a healthy way.

MYTH 5: ADULTS CANNOT DO ANYTHING TO HELP YOUNG PERFECTIONISTS

The frustration of parents and teachers dealing with perfectionism among children can be heard in almost any town, school, or neighborhood. Often, adults do not know where to turn or what to do to help their young children exhibiting unhealthy perfectionism. The goal of these adults is to change the negative aspects of unhealthy perfectionism into healthier habits. Fortunately, researchers in psychology and education have developed strategies and interventions to help perfectionists use their perfectionism in a healthy way.

What the Research Says

Interventions and therapy procedures have been developed for psychologists and trained therapists to use with children to address unhealthy perfectionism. These range from highly formal and structured formats to more flexible formats. For example, one researcher used an online forum to connect students with perfectionism and give them opportunities to reflect on their thought processes (Aldea, 2008).

One popular intervention with positive results in the research is **cognitive behavior therapy**. Cognitive behavior therapy focuses on adjusting the negative thought patterns, assumptions, beliefs, evaluations, and behaviors of people into more positive and healthy outcomes. This therapy has been shown to reduce unhealthy perfectionism as well as depression and anxiety (Arpin-Cribbie, 2008). It has been used with patients in a clinical setting (Riley, Lee, Cooper, Fairburn, & Shafran, 2007), as well as in nonclinical settings (Kearns, Forbes, & Gardiner, 2007; Keans, Gardiner, & Marshall, 2008).

Another strategy used with younger children is **play therapy**, in which therapists employ an interpersonal environment to evaluate and modify a child's behavior and cognitions. Popular strategies in play therapy include:

- ▶ helping the child identify negative themes within his or her play,
- ▶ providing ways for the child to cope with mistakes and criticism,
- ▶ expanding the child's choices for play materials,
- ▶ helping the child cope with anxiety, and
- ▶ helping the child develop a greater tolerance for mistakes (Ashby et al., 2004).

Play therapy advocates also suggest games that do not have a clear winner, such as the Ungame or Sleeping Grump (Ashby et al., 2004; see Chapter 11 for a description of these games). Studies have shown that play therapy may be very effective for overcoming perfectionism in children (Ashby et al., 2004; Daigneault, 1999).

If the child's perfectionism affects his or her health and well-being, be sure to seek professional help.

Other strategies include the development of **coping resources** to help children move from unhealthy to healthy perfectionism. The possession of these coping resources have been identified as one difference between students with healthy and unhealthy perfectionism (Nounopoulos, Ashby, & Gilman, 2006; Stoltz & Ashby, 2007). These coping resources include the following (Nounopoulos et al., 2006):

- **social confidence**, or how able a child is able to disclose his or her feelings and opinions in social settings;
- **behavior control**, or how well a child is able to cooperate with others;
- **academic confidence**, or how much confidence the child has in his or her ability to do well in school and produce quality work;
- **peer acceptance**, or how much the student is accepted by classmates; and
- **family support,** the degree of support from family.

Helping students to develop these coping resources may help students to overcome unhealthy perfectionism and to use their perfectionism in a positive manner.

Final Thoughts

Although many teachers and parents may still be searching for help with their perfectionistic children, there is help available. If the issues surrounding a child's perfectionism seem to be debilitating and interfering with a child's life, then professional help through psychologists or trained therapists is available. These therapies may include cognitive behavior therapy, play therapy, and coaching in coping resources. Parents and teachers may work with these professionals to help children develop healthy perfectionism in the place of unhealthy behaviors. In addition to these techniques, many of which have been documented through research, many parents have found success in holistic therapy and meditation exercises, such as yoga.

MYTH 6: THERE IS ONLY ONE TYPE OF PERFECTIONIST

Teachers and parents tend to categorize students as either perfectionists or nonperfectionists. In this conception, all perfectionists fit the same set of characteristics and are marked by similar behaviors, motivations, and outcomes. However, research suggests that perfectionism can be categorized by many different variables (i.e., Dixon, Lapsley, & Hanchon, 2004). We have already discussed the differences between healthy and unhealthy perfectionism. In addition, various researchers have conceptualized perfectionism in other terms.

What the Research Says

Unhealthy, healthy, and **nonperfectionism** are ways to categorize perfectionistic behaviors. This model of categorization focuses on the positive and negative aspects of perfectionism. Other researchers have identified three other categories: self-oriented, other-oriented, and socially prescribed perfectionism (Blankstein, Lumley, & Crawford, 2007; Speirs Neumeister, 2004). **Self-oriented perfectionism** is characterized by a strong sense of self-motivation. In this type of perfectionism, the child holds him- or herself to extremely high standards. **Other-oriented perfectionism** is when a child holds other people to high standards and perfection. **Socially prescribed perfectionism** is when a child believes that other people hold him or her to high standards and are critical of his or her mistakes. Each of these types of perfectionism may be either healthy or unhealthy. Table 4 describes characteristics of these three types of perfectionists.

Perfectionists vary in whom they hold high expectations for and for whom they are trying to be perfect.

Table 4

Types of Perfectionism

Self-Oriented Perfectionism	Self-motivated, the child holds him- or herself to extremely high standards
Other-Oriented Perfectionism	Focused on others, the child holds others to high standards
Socially Prescribed Perfectionism	Focused on others, the child believes others hold him or her to high standards

Final Thoughts

In addition to these models, we have observed other patterns of perfectionism in children. We have classified these behaviors into the following categories: the Academic Achiever, the Aggravated Accuracy Assessor, the Risk Evader, the Controlling Image Manager, and the Procrastinating Perfectionist. Table 5 describes each category briefly, delineating a few characteristics of each. These categories are not exclusive of one another. Rather, they capture general perfectionistic behaviors that may be used in a healthy or unhealthy manner. Each of these profiles will be discussed in further detail in the following chapters.

MYTH 7: PERFECTIONISM IS NOT REALLY THAT HARMFUL FOR CHILDREN

Parents and teachers view perfectionism as a problem and issue for children, but they sometimes underestimate the seriousness of perfectionism for some students. This can be particularly true for gifted children, who have such high capabilities that their perfectionism may seem to "pay off," or result in high achievement. Unhealthy

Table 5

Profiles of Perfectionists

Academic Achievers 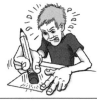	Hold unrealistically high expectations for their performance in academic pursuits; focus on the final grade and on mistakes made
Aggravated Accuracy Assessors 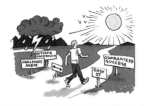	May choose to redo the same work over and over to try to make it more like their mind's ideal; may look frantically for ways to "fix" their work or find the necessary materials; may become disappointed and give up trying
Risk Evaders 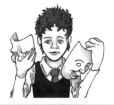	Fear failure to achieve their standards and ideals due to asynchronous development or physical limitations; choose not to attempt the task
Controlling Image Managers 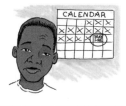	Want others to regard them as perfect; if they are afraid they are unable to meet expectations in competitive situations, choose to eliminate themselves intentionally and say they *could have* been perfect if they wanted to compete
Procrastinating Perfectionists	Plan an extensive project but fail to start it for fear of their inability to achieve their perfect vision

Note. From Adelson (2007).

manifestations of perfectionism often are seen as an issue that has only short-term, not long-term, consequences for students. Thus, parents and teachers sometimes ignore perfectionism in children. However, research suggests that unhealthy perfectionism may be closely associated with many more serious problems for children and lead to larger forms of **psychological distress**.

What the Research Says

Several studies have shown that unhealthy perfectionism tends to increase over time (Kline & Short, 1991; Siegle & Schuler, 2000; Waller, Wood, Miller, & Slade, 1992). This indicates a need to intervene early in a child's life in order to avoid later escalation of unhealthy perfectionism. The negative aspects of perfectionism have been documented in many studies as well, and range from severity of headaches (Kowal & Pritchard, 1990), social anxiety (Biran & Reese, 2007; Laurenti, Bruch, & Haase, 2008), greater levels of anger among athletes (Vallance, Dunn, & Dunn, 2006), and poor health and greater alcohol consumption in college (Pritchard, Wilson, & Yamnitz, 2007).

Early intervention is important to help perfectionists use their perfectionism in a healthy way.

Much of the research concerning unhealthy perfectionism is linked to eating disorders (Chang, Ivezaj, Downey, Kashima, & Morady, 2008). Children and adolescents who view perfection as the ideal goal often turn those expectations not only to academics but also to their body image. Unhealthy perfectionism has been linked to greater severity of **anorexia** (Castro-Fornieles et al., 2007; Waller et al., 1992) and **bulimia** (Bardone-Cone, 2007; Castro-Fornieles et al.; Downey & Chang, 2007). Interestingly, socially prescribed perfectionism is more closely associated with bulimia, while self-oriented perfectionism is linked to anorexia (Brannan & Petrie,

2008). However it should be noted that some studies have found that perfectionism is not necessarily predictive of later eating disorders (Calam & Waller, 1998). For further information on this subject, see the resources listed in Chapter 11.

Unhealthy perfectionism also is linked to psychological distress, including anxiety and depression (Hewitt et al., 2002). For instance, unhealthy perfectionism is associated with higher levels of depression in children (Flamenbaum & Holden, 2007; Huprich, Porcerelli, Keaschuk, Binienda, & Engle, 2008; Jones, 2008; Leon, Kendall, & Garber, 1980) and greater levels of fatigue (Arpin-Cribbie & Cribbie, 2007). Links between unhealthy perfectionism and symptoms of anxiety (Dekryger, 2006) include excessive worry (Chang et al., 2007). Again, for further information on this subject, see the resources listed in Chapter 11.

Finally, unhealthy perfectionism and the associated anxiety and depression can lead to suicide and suicidal thoughts in children and adolescents (O'Connor, 2007). Socially prescribed perfectionism seems to be most identified with suicidal thoughts and suicide attempts (Blankstein et al., 2007; Boergers, Spirito, & Donaldson, 1998; Hewitt, Newton, Flett, & Callander, 1997). Obviously, any mention of suicidal thoughts or indications of possible suicidal behavior should be brought to trained psychologists, counselors, or therapists, in any situation.

Final Thoughts

Unhealthy perfectionism should not be taken lightly by parents or teachers. Although the symptoms may seem minor in early childhood, these behaviors may escalate throughout the years and lead to more serious psychological consequences. These consequences may include anxiety, depression, and eating disorders. Teachers and parents can intervene when they see unhealthy perfectionism and help guide children toward healthier cognitive processes and behaviors. When the symptoms lead to greater psychological distress or debilitating behaviors, parents and teachers should contact professional counselors, psychologists, or therapists for more intensive interventions.

SUMMARY

Many parents and teachers hold misconceptions about perfectionism. Through a careful review of the relevant research concerning perfectionism, many of these myths can be dispelled. This chapter has summarized the major research about perfectionism and provided information relevant to both parents and teachers concerning the children in their lives.

3

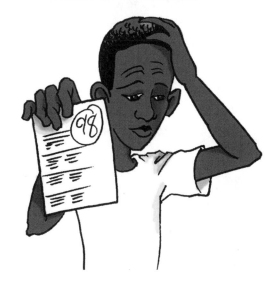

THE ACADEMIC ACHIEVER

"Must Achieve 100%"

Caroline, a fourth grader, was a strong math student. Her teacher was working with her on sixth-grade mathematics content. She came home one night, and when her parents asked how her day at school was, she burst into tears. Once she calmed down, she explained that she had "failed a math test" and was too upset to explain. The next day, her parents stopped by the school to talk to Caroline's teacher. The test she had "failed" was a diagnostic test (a pretest). When they sat down with Caroline, she explained that she felt that she couldn't leave any answers blank—she had to know how to solve it or she wasn't smart in math. Despite the diagnostic nature of the assessment, Caroline struggled with the idea of skipping a problem and of struggling to solve a problem, whether she ever had been exposed to the concepts being tested or not.

Eric, another student talented in math, always came home and did his math homework first thing. He would do the assigned problems and then ask his parents to check them. If he missed even one due to a "careless" error, he believed he did not know the material well enough and would do numerous additional problems. Even after he had mastered a concept or skill, he often would continue to practice and feel insecure in his abilities because he did not do perfectly on the practice.

Shawanda's teacher had a policy that if the students misspelled no more than one word on the spelling pretest, then they did not have to take the test at the end of the week. However, when Shawanda missed a word, she came home upset at her performance and studied her words. Her parents assumed that she had to take the posttest since Shawanda studied

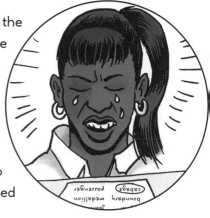

the words and did the spelling homework every night. They did not realize that this was her own decision because she felt she was not perfect on the pretest.

Kalon's class was reviewing what they had learned over the course of the year in social studies in preparation for the state test. Although Kalon had a firm grasp of the concepts and key ideas that they had studied, he expected himself to remember every detail about each person, place, or event. During a review game, he knew the answer to the final question but did not remember exactly how it had been worded on his review sheet. He started pounding his head, trying to remember, and even after he won the game (and received credit for providing the correct answer to the final question), he sat frustrated with himself trying to remember the precise wording.

Kwan's family moved from Korea to the United States when he was in kindergarten. Prior to that, Kwan had not been exposed to English. Later in elementary school, Kwan was identified for the self-contained gifted and talented class and worked very hard to earn top grades. He was particularly interested in mathematics and science, which both came easily to him. By fourth grade, Kwan was reading above grade level. However, his grade point average in language arts was a low A. His parents worried about his reading ability and would request extra assignments for him. Moreover, Kwan was distraught about his language arts grade and believed he "wasn't good" at reading.

Blair loved to write poetry. She had been reading poetry since she had learned to read,
and as a third grader, she had several
notebooks filled with her poems. During recess, she often would sit under the
slide and write. When the PTA had an
arts competition, Blair decided to write a
poem for the entry. She worked every day
on writing a poem to match the theme, and
she finally had a poem she was happy with and
excitedly submitted it. The day of the PTA program, she hopefully
waited to hear the awards. However, she was crestfallen when they
announced she had won second place. She went home after the
program, threw away her notebooks, and told her parents she would
never write a poem again because she was not good at it.

Academic Achievers are academically oriented students who
exhibit negative perfectionism in their academic pursuits. They hold
unrealistically high expectations for their own academic performance
and expect perfection, and nothing less, from themselves. Typically,
these students are high achievers with high grades, but they become
disappointed with themselves when they earn anything less than a
perfect score. They often are not satisfied with the achievements and
grades they earn, wanting to earn all of the extra credit points possible
and wanting to know the highest possible score for each **assessment**.
Even when they earn high grades, Academic Achievers are not satisfied with a "100" on an assignment or test, regularly completing extra
credit projects and assignments with as much energy and effort as

they put into their required work to score the maximum number of points possible.

Often, the identity of Academic Achievers lies in their academic achievements, and they see a mistake as a sign of failure and a flaw in their identity. Academic Achievers become very frustrated with themselves if they do not earn the top grade or cannot remember an answer "word-for-word" on every formal and informal assessment. Putting forth effort in their schoolwork typically is not an issue for Academic Achievers.

In fact, due to the extremely high standards that they impose on themselves, Academic Achievers often put forth more effort than required to master the material and achieve at the top level. Rather than a lack of effort being a problem, they sometimes have a problem with being too fixated on putting effort into perfecting something rather than moving on to the next subject, problem, or challenge. Homework can be a struggle for these students as they see every assessment—**informal** or **formal**, **summative** or **formative**—as an evaluation of their intelligence and their self-worth. They do not see practice or homework as an opportunity to learn and to improve. Similarly, they have trouble understanding the purpose of **diagnostic** tests and believe their inability to answer a question or to solve a problem means they are "not smart" or a failure. When taught a new concept or skill, Academic Achievers expect to immediately be proficient and demonstrate mastery without mistakes. They do not take pleasure in the struggles of a difficult problem and cannot experience the joy of an "Aha!" moment because they often become frustrated with themselves and give up easily when faced with a new academic challenge. They see the challenge

Academic Achievers often have identities tightly tied to their academic achievement. Thus, imperfect achievement at school may lead to **imposter syndrome**.

not as an opportunity to grow and learn but as a testament to their own failure and flaws.

Another issue for Academic Achievers is their tendency to focus heavily on their mistakes. Even when they meet the expectations of the task at hand, these students, unfortunately, rarely are satisfied with their performance. Rather than looking at the progress or the process, Academic Achievers are focused on the end product, particularly on the evaluation of that product (typically a grade), and they judge themselves on that criteria alone. They might come home and express to their parents that they "failed" a test because it was challenging or because they earned a low A or a B. They fixate on imperfect grades on a report card or on the handful of questions they may have missed on a test. Because their identity is tied to their academic achievements, if they are in an academic competition, including review games in the classroom, they can become distraught and believe they are "dumb" if they do not win. Missing one question out of a hundred might result in crumpled papers and tears rather than satisfaction in correctly answering 99% of the questions or in improving from the previous test. For Academic Achievers, mistakes are glaring, and success is defined by perfection.

Although the pressure for perfect work often is internal for Academic Achievers, who tie their identity to their academic achievements, this pressure also can arise from the expectations of family and peers. In some cases, like that of Kwan, family pressures feed the Academic Achiever's stress on him- or herself for perfection. A parent's focus on doing well academically and on achieving specific grades might fuel an Academic Achiever's own internal pressure to do well. Additionally, being referred to as "The Smart One" in a family or group or being consistently praised for being "so smart" and getting all A's, might create further tension in the Academic

Academic Achievers are overly focused on their mistakes and not their successes and mastery of concepts.

Achiever because it solidifies the academically oriented identity that is tied to the child's outcomes and to process or progress. The label of "gifted" or being pulled out for special programs may create a similar atmosphere for students. This internal identity for the Academic Achiever often is furthered by comments made by parents, siblings, other relatives, peers, or the teacher. Although these people may not be disappointed with less than perfection, Academic Achievers might believe they are letting these people down and cannot make academic mistakes or admit not knowing something.

STRATEGIES FOR THE CLASSROOM

Because the Academic Achiever's identity is so tied into his or her academic achievement, it is essential that educators are aware of these students in their classrooms. Although it is easy and quite natural for educators and parents alike to praise students for high grades, it is more important for you to praise students, particularly Academic Achievers, for their efforts and progress. Rather than focusing on "being smart" and earning good grades, you need to place significantly more emphasis on the effort and **problem-solving strategies** of Academic Achievers. This becomes a model for students, but it is not enough. Academic Achievers need guidance from their teachers in how to take pride in the process and how to use mistakes as learning experiences. **Diagnostic assessments**, or tests used at the beginning of units of study to determine the knowledge students already possess on a topic, are not only tools for acceleration and com-

> **Successful Strategies for the Classroom**
> ► Praise for efforts and progress
> ► Use diagnostic testing and focus on growth
> ► Use formative assessment as a tool to teach learning from mistakes
> ► Use portfolios and reflection to help students recognize strengths
> ► Incorporate practice on students' weaknesses into topics or areas of strength

pacting, but also good tools for working with Academic Achievers. These types of assessment can teach them not to expect perfection on everything academic in nature, teaching them that assessments can be formative as well as summative. For example, after Caroline's teacher worked with her on identifying areas of strengths and weaknesses, she learned the purpose of diagnostic testing and learned to take them with less anxiety, eagerly helping to pinpoint the content and skills she did not know.

Academic Achievers are focused on summative evaluation and on the final grade, without an eye toward learning from mistakes. Besides using formative assessment for your own purposes, you also should use it as an opportunity to guide students in learning from their mistakes and recognizing their own mastery. To help Eric focus more on learning from his mistakes rather than only despairing at his imperfections, his teacher asked him to correct his mistakes and write **"WIMI's"** (**"Why I Missed It"**; see Chapter 9) statements. This approach removed the emphasis from "less than 100%" to learning from mistakes and recognizing reasons Eric incorrectly solved problems. Eric came to recognize that mastery and perfection were not equivalent and that practice helps us learn from our mistakes but does not need to be perfect.

Similarly, once Shawanda's teacher met with her parents and they realized what Shawanda was doing, they worked with her on not penalizing herself for not being perfect. Rather than focusing on the entire list during the week, Shawanda's teacher would allow her to spell the one word she missed during the posttest, focusing the attention on learning from her pretest and accepting mastery of the other words. After a few weeks, Shawanda realized that when she misspelled a word, she still had mastered the list for that week and no longer participated in the posttest. Instead, she would study words from a challenge list so that she could compete in the district spelling bee later that year.

In addition to learning from their mistakes, Academic Achievers need to learn to recognize their improvement and progress rather than basing their evaluation on a final grade or assessment. For Kalon, who was so focused on achievement that he had to remember everything word-for-word, seeing his growth in understanding helped him not be so hard on himself and have such unrealistic expectations. At the beginning of a unit, Kalon's teacher had him create a concept map showing what he already knew about the topic. As part of his final assessment, Kalon created another concept map or **mind map** to demonstrate his additional learning. Comparing the two, Kalon had a visual representation that allowed him to see that he truly had learned a lot and to focus more on concepts rather than precise wording. For Blair, whose focus was on the final evaluation, her teacher worked with her on critiquing her poetry that she submitted to competitions and keeping a poetry portfolio. In her critique, Blair learned to identify the strengths of her poetry, as well as look at it from the eye of a judge on what could be improved. More than that, with each submission, Blair took some time to review her portfolio and list improvements in her poetry. This helped her enjoy competitions more as she could take pride in her improvements, which were under her control, rather than focus on how she did compared to others.

Recognizing improvement and progress sometimes is not enough. Some Academic Achievers, like Kwan, are so focused on their weaknesses that they do not recognize, much less celebrate, their strengths. Kwan continued to work on his language arts skills, but his teacher worked with him to move the focus from the grade to improvement, keeping a portfolio and reflecting on progress throughout the year. Rather than focusing solely on his "weakness" and comparing it to the abilities of his peers, Kwan needed to begin recognizing his strengths. His teacher met with him at the beginning of each marking period to discuss his strengths, his improvements, and what he would like to achieve during the next marking period. Moreover, she used recommended best practices and helped Kwan address his "weakness" though his strengths—incorporating more reading and writing in Kwan's mathematics and science assignments, which piqued his interest and helped him to improve.

STRATEGIES FOR THE HOME

Parents of Academic Achievers often find themselves in awkward situations. On one hand, they are pleased with their child's commitment to academic success, but on the other hand, they are troubled by their child's sometimes unhealthy obsession with perfection in academic tasks. It may be difficult for parents to find support from other parents or school personnel and resources for their situation.

One step that you can take is to focus family goals less on grades and more on academic learning. This may be accomplished through careful observation of the words used with children when discussing school. For example, you may ask what the child learned from a project or from a unit of study, rather than what grade he or she obtained on the final product or chapter test. You may even want to avoid looking at report cards and grades in front of your child, focusing instead on listening to your child discuss his or her learning and accomplishments. If your child already is aware of his or her grades, then, in most situations, it is unnecessary for you to place additional emphasis on grades. Instead, you should focus on areas that your child improved and also talk about strategies for your child to improve any areas that he or she is not pleased with.

Successful Strategies for the Home
- De-emphasize grades
- Celebrate learning and growth
- Be an example in your mistakes
- Choose books and movies to illustrate "flawed protagonists"
- Find off-peak times to talk to your child

Instead of focusing on the teacher's and others' evaluations of student achievement, you should celebrate your child's learning and growth. Family dinners, car rides to and from school activities, and other moments provide excellent opportunities to discuss with your child his or her achievements for the day that are separated from others' evaluations of those activities. You can work with your child during these times to feel pride in learning a new skill in math, rather than focusing his or her pride on an A on the final test. The goal here is to move your child from relying on **extrinsic rewards**, such as grades, to **intrinsic rewards**, such as the feeling of accomplishment from learning a new skill.

To extend this idea, your family may wish to have a celebration at the end of each unit of study, grading period, or semester to recognize the accomplishments of each family member. These accomplishments should not be external evaluations of accomplishment. Rather, they should focus on the growth and learning that took place during the time period. One family, for example, ordered pizza and had ice cream at the end of each grading period. During the course of the meal, each family member, parents included, shared the area in which he or she felt he or she had learned the most during the 6-week time period. Another family chose to celebrate each time a family member completed a significant project. This celebration occurred before feedback from the teacher, or supervisor, was given, keeping the focus on the accomplishment that the family member felt at completing the task. This helped to emphasize the internal rewards of working hard at a project, rather than the external evaluation from others. Additionally, if your child has taken a pre- and posttest on a topic, you can use that to help your child recognize and celebrate growth made during the course of a unit of study.

When struggling with an Academic Achiever, many parents look toward biographies, books, and movies for examples that show a healthy balance of success and failures. Even notable figures did not perform perfectly on every occasion. Albert Einstein missed key questions on his college entrance exams. And, although Mary Lou Retton won the gold All-Around medal in the 1984 Olympics, she only won the bronze on the floor exercise. See the following list (Figure 1) from a leading researcher of the social and emotional needs of gifted children for some other possible biographies. This list originally was created for use with gifted teenagers, but could apply to many middle school students' interests; however, parents and teachers of younger students may wish to read or look over some of the titles before using them. Children also may wish to research their own heroes and heroines to find out about not only their successes but times at which they were less than perfect.

Educators are familiar with the term **"teachable moment,"** in which an unexpected event in the classroom provides an excellent opportunity to extend student learning. As a parent, you can look for similar moments when you are with your children, whether they are watching TV, going to the movies, or reading the newspaper. Characters in sitcoms often make mistakes, but part of the lesson of the show is for the character to admit his or her mistake and move on. This type of situation may need to be emphasized to children and talked about in a family discussion. Parents also can observe their children's interactions with other children carefully; peer interactions can offer multiple teaching moments to apply simple situations like board games or craft projects to the idea of general improvement or completion of a task as opposed to being the best or winning in a competitive situation.

"The most important tool for parents is communication with their children."

In addition to teachable moments, many parents find success talking with children about delicate situations, such as unhealthy perfectionism, during **"off-peak times."** Off-peak times are times at which the situation is not immediately pressing and both parents and children are calm. For example, you

Biographies of Women of Achievement

- **Madeleine Albright** (Secretary of State)

    Albright, M. (2003). *Madam secretary: A memoir.* New York: Hyperion Books.

    Dobbs, M. (1999). *Madeleine Albright: A twentieth century odyssey.* New York: Holt.

- **Maya Angelou** (Author and Poet)

    Angelou, M. (1969). *I know why the caged bird sings.* New York: Bantam Books.

- **Melba Pattillo Beals** (Author and Journalist)

    Beals, M. P. (1994). *Warriors don't cry: A searing memoir of the battle to integrate Little Rock's Central High.* New York: Washington Square Press.

- **Rachel Carson** (Environmentalist)

    Lear, L. (1997). *Rachel Carson: Witness for nature.* New York: Henry Holt.

- **Sandra Cisneros** (Author)

    Mirriam-Goldberg, C. (1998). *Sandra Cisneros: Latina writer and activist.* Springfield, NJ: Enslow.

- **Amelia Earhart** (Pilot)

    Butler, S. (1997). *East to dawn: The life of Amelia Earhart.* Reading, MA: Addison-Wesley.

- **Lorraine Hansberry** (Playwright)

    Hansberry, L. (1969). *To be young, gifted and Black: An informal autobiography of Lorraine Hansberry.* New York: Penguin.

- **Leta Hollingworth** (Educator)

    Klein, A. (2002). *A forgotten voice: A biography of Leta Stetter Hollingworth.* Scottsdale, AZ: Great Potential Press.

- **Barbara Jordan** (Politician)

    Rogers, M. (1998). *Barbara Jordan: An American hero.* New York: Bantam.

- **Helen Keller** (Author and Activist)

    Keller, H. (2003). *The story of my life.* New York: W. W. Norton & Company.

- **Coretta Scott King** (Human Rights Activist)

    Vivian, O. (2006). *Coretta: The story of Coretta Scott King.* Minneapolis, MN: Fortress Press.

- **Wilma Mankiller** (Leader of the Cherokee Nation)

    Mankiller, W. (1993). *Wilma Mankiller: A chief and her people.* New York: St. Martin's Press.

Figure 1. Biographies suggested for use with gifted teenagers.

Note. Adapted from Hébert (2009). Adapted with permission.

- **Sandra Day O'Connor** (Supreme Court Justice)
  Biskupic, J. (2005). *Sandra Day O'Connor: How the first woman on the Supreme Court became its most influential justice.* New York: Harper Perennial.
  Day O'Connor, S., & Day, A. (2002). *Lazy B: Growing up on a cattle ranch in the American southwest.* New York: Random House.
- **Mary Lou Retton** (Athlete)
  Retton, M. L. (2000). *Mary Lou Retton's gateways to happiness.* New York: Broadway Books.
- **Condoleezza Rice** (Secretary of State)
  Felix, A. (2002). *Condi: The Condoleezza Rice story.* New York: Newmarket Press.
- **Esmerelda Santiago** (Author and Screenwriter)
  Santiago, E. (1993). *When I was Puerto Rican.* New York: Vintage.
  Santiago, E. (1998). *Almost a Woman.* New York: Vintage.
- **Beverly Sills** (Opera Singer)
  Sills, B. (1976). *Bubbles: A self-portrait.* New York: Bobbs-Merrill.
  Sills, B., & Linderman, L. (1987). *Beverly: An autobiography.* New York: Bantam Books.
- **Maria Tallchief** (Ballerina)
  Tallchief, M. (1997). *Maria Tallchief: America's prima ballerina.* New York: Holt.
- **Heather Whitestone** (Miss America, Motivational Speaker)
  Gray, D. (1995). *Yes, you can, Heather!* Grand Rapids, MI: Zondervan.
  Whitestone, H., & Hunt, A. (1998). *Listening with my heart.* New York: Doubleday.

Biographies of Men of Achievement

- **Neil Armstrong** (Astronaut)
  Hansen, J. (2005). *First man: The life of Neil A. Armstrong.* New York: Simon & Schuster.
- **Russell Baker** (Author)
  Baker, R. (1982). *Growing up.* New York: Congdon & Weed.
- **Tom Brokaw** (Television Journalist)
  Brokaw, T. (2002). *A long way from home: Growing up in the American heartland.* New York: Random House.
- **Jim Carrey** (Actor)
  Knelman, M. (2000). *Jim Carrey: The joker is wild.* Buffalo, NY: Firefly Books.

Figure 1, Continued

- **Ben Carson** (Surgeon)

   Carson, B. (1990). *Gifted hands: The Ben Carson story.* Grand Rapids, MI: Zondervan.

   Carson, B., & Murphy, C. (1992). *Think big: Unleashing your potential for excellence.* Grand Rapids, MI: Zondervan.

- **Jimmy Carter** (President)

   Carter, J. (2001). *An hour before daylight: Memories of a rural boyhood.* New York: Simon & Schuster.

- **Anderson Cooper** (Television Journalist)

   Cooper, A. (2006). *Dispatches from the edge: A memoir of war, disasters, and survival.* New York: HarperCollins.

- **Bill Gates** (Entrepreneur)

   Manes, S., & Andrews, P. (1994). *Gates.* New York: Simon & Schuster.

   Wallace, J., & Erickson, J. (1992). *Hard drive: Bill Gates and the making of the Microsoft empire.* New York: John Wiley & Sons.

- **John Glenn** (Astronaut)

   Glenn, J., & Taylor, N. (1999). *John Glenn: A memoir.* New York: Bantam Books.

- **Tony Hawk** (Athlete)

   Hawk, T., & Mortimer, S. (2000). *Hawk: Occupation: Skateboarder.* New York: HarperCollins.

- **Homer Hickam, Jr.** (Aerospace Engineer)

   Hickam, H., Jr. (1998). *October sky.* New York: Dell.

- **Michael Jordan** (Athlete)

   Greene, B. (1992). *Hang time: Days and dreams with Michael Jordan.* New York: St. Martin's Press.

- **Martin Luther King, Jr.** (Civil Rights Leader)

   Carson, C. (Ed.). (1998). *The autobiography of Martin Luther King, Jr.* New York: Warner.

- **Carl Lewis** (Athlete)

   Lewis, C. (1990). *Inside track: My professional life in amateur track and field.* New York: Simon & Schuster.

- **John McCain** (Politician)

   McCain, J. (1999). *Faith of my fathers.* New York: Random House.

- **Ruben Navarette** (Journalist)

   Navarette, R., Jr. (1993). *A darker shade of crimson: Odyssey of a Harvard Chicano.* New York: Bantam.

- **Barack Obama** (President)

   Obama, B. (2004). *Dreams from my father: A story of race and inheritance.* New York: Three Rivers Press.

Figure 1, Continued

- **Colin Powell** (Secretary of State)
  DeYoung, K. (2006). *Soldier: The life of Colin Powell.* New York: Alfred A. Knopf.
  Powell, C. (1995). *My American journey.* New York: Random House.
  Steins, R. (2003). *Colin Powell: A biography.* Westport, CT: Greenwood Press.
- **Dan Rather** (Television Journalist)
  Rather, D. (1991). *I remember.* Boston: Little, Brown.
  Weisman, A. (2006). *Lone star: The extraordinary life and times of Dan Rather.* Hoboken, NJ: John Wiley & Sons.
- **Richard Rodriguez** (Journalist)
  Rodriguez, R. (1982). *Hunger of memory: The education of Richard Rodriguez.* New York: Bantam.
  Rodriguez, R. (1992). *Days of obligation: An argument with my Mexican father.* New York: Viking.
  Rodriguez, R. (2002). *Brown: The last discovery of America.* New York: Penguin.
- **Tim Russert** (Television Journalist)
  Russert, T. (2004). *Big Russ & me: Father and son—Lessons of life.* New York: Miramax.
- **Carlos Santana** (Musician)
  Shapiro, M. (2000). *Carlos Santana: Back on top.* New York: St. Martin's Press.
- **Steven Spielberg** (Film Director)
  McBride, J. (1997). *Steven Spielberg: A biography.* New York: Simon & Schuster.

may experience more success in talking with your child about perfectionism, not when your child is in the middle of a breakdown but at a time when your child is not necessarily thinking about schoolwork, such as on the ride home from soccer practice or when you are cuddling up with a good book at bedtime.

Although the parents of Academic Achievers often find the situation overwhelming and frustrating, there are several strategies that may help their child have a healthy balance of academic endeavors as noted above. The most important tool for parents is communication with their children. By communicating about expectations and how we define learning and success, you can help your child set reasonable academic goals and standards and focus on growing as a learner.

FINAL THOUGHTS

Academic Achievers hold themselves to unrealistically high expectations in academic endeavors. They easily can become fixated on anything less than a perfect score. They do not see the goals of education as being to improve, to learn, and to master new content and skills. Instead, they expect to know everything on the first attempt and see all academic activities as something they must complete flawlessly. Parents and teachers of Academic Achievers can work with them to change their unrealistic expectations into realistic goals, focusing on personal growth rather than perfection.

4

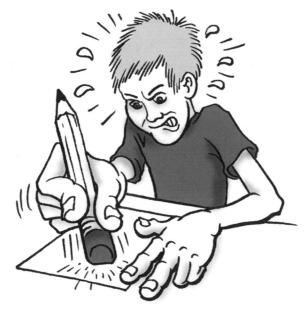

THE AGGRAVATED ACCURACY ASSESSOR

"Exactness and Fixation on 'Redos'"

Ivan exhibited artistic talent at a young age. He was particularly talented at drawing portraits, creating realistic drawings that were quite precise given his age (fourth grade) and still-developing fine motor skills. The fourth graders were creating paintings for a Virginia studies art gallery in their school, and Ivan had decided to draw a

Confederate soldier. During several art classes, Ivan meticulously worked on his drawing. He would tune out all of his classmates and be completely absorbed in the fine details of his drawing. His concentration was broken by only one thing—he constantly would get up and take the drawing to the art teacher and his classroom teacher for reassurance that it was "good." Every time Ivan's drawing neared completion, he would decide to redo the drawing because it was not precise enough. He would see some detail that was not just right and crumple up the drawing, starting over.

By the time children are in upper elementary school, they are beginning to learn to take notes in class. Many students appreciate this opportunity to use shorthand, not to worry so much about handwriting, and not to be expected to create a "final copy." However, Leta dreaded any time she had to take notes in class because she just did not have enough time for preciseness. In fifth grade, Leta's social studies teacher was working with the students on different note-taking strategies, and her class was followed immediately by recess. Each day that they worked on note taking, when the other students excitedly went out to play, Leta would ask to stay and continue writing or copying her notes. She would painstakingly write each individual letter of every word, taking extra time and putting forth extra effort to ensure that her notes were as neat as possible. If given the opportunity, Leta would rewrite her notes, not as a method of learning the material but because she was frustrated at how "messy" they were. At times, Leta would fall behind in another class because she was fixated on rewriting her notes or finishing her notes and could not mentally or physically move on to another subject. Her mom found her homework taking her much longer than would be expected at this age and realized that Leta was bringing her notebooks home and recopying everything, sometimes erasing so many times to make each individual letter perfect that she would rip a hole in the paper, creating a meltdown because she then had to start all over again. Her mother often was left bewildered and frustrated as a result of Leta's meltdowns.

Devon, a third grader, was interested in architecture. From a young age, he had been fascinated with the different types of buildings related to the cultures and time periods his teachers would introduce to the class. When studying ancient Egypt, he decided to build a replica of a pyramid. He carefully researched the architecture and design of the interior, the dimensions, the materials, and all other aspects of the Great Pyramids before he began gathering his materials and creating his pyramid. He would spend several hours working on the pyramid, make substantial progress, and then decide that some angle was not "just right" or a dimension was too short or too long and would start all over. The school's Open House took place almost one month after Devon had started building his pyramid. His parents came and saw the projects that Devon's classmates had been working on and mostly had finished. However, when they asked Devon where his pyramid was, he showed them the plans for his pyramid. He did not have anything built at that point because he had, once again, decided to start over from the beginning.

Andy had been skateboarding almost as long as he had been walking. He loved the sport, and he would spend as much time as possible at the local skate park. He was in fifth grade, and he already was competing in skate contests and holding his own against competitors 4 to 7 years older than him. He would watch videos of professional skaters like Tony Hawk and Bob Burnquist, memorizing every trick that they did. Andy's favorite trick was the Ollie 540, and he would use his TV's slow motion capability to watch the skaters' form and movements as they completed the trick. However, he could not do the trick himself. He would spend hours, until well past exhaustion, working on the same move over and over. One problem that Andy had was that he was going through a growth spurt and was experiencing awkward coordination as he "grew into" his body. He also had yet to master some of the skills leading up to this level of trick. Despite these limitations, he insisted he knew how to do it and refused to stop practicing it, often to the detriment of his schoolwork and the development of other skateboarding skills.

Radhika loved the piano. She had been playing for several years and thoroughly enjoyed both competing and practicing. Her parents did not have to encourage her to practice—she did so on her own, often longer than her instructor had suggested she had to each day. On more than one occasion, Radhika would turn down an invitation to play with her friends because she was in the middle of practicing. Radhika had chosen a particularly difficult piece to play for an upcoming concert. Although she had picked the piece well in advance, the concert was only a week away, and she still had not played the piece all the way through. Radhika would get a little ways into the piece, make an error—whether playing a wrong key, holding a note too long, or even forgetting to change volumes immediately—and would get frustrated and start again from the beginning. She refused to continue the song after making any mistake; therefore, she had yet to practice the second half of the song at all. In her lessons, the instructor sometimes would not even hear the error, but Radhika would stop, frustrated with herself for not being perfect. When pushed to continue she would become so perturbed about not being perfect that she would lose her concentration and fumble through the rest of the song, often bringing herself to tears. At one point, she declared she just could not do it any more and refused to play the rest of the song.

Trisha had been working on her tessellation project for her mathematics class for 2 weeks. Her mom had asked her several times to see her work, but Trisha always told her it wasn't ready yet. Whenever her mom came to her room while she was working on the tessellation, Trisha would quickly hide her work. She kept telling her mom that she had to fix it, that it wasn't just right yet, and that she would show her when it was perfect.

The night before the project was due, Trisha's mom again asked to see the project. Trisha again said it wasn't ready and asked if she could start over. When her mom explained that it was getting late and due the next day, Trisha frantically searched for a large eraser and White-Out and ran back to her room. Her mom found her in there trying to edit her work completely. When she asked Trisha what she was doing, Trisha explained that she just had to fix it—no matter what she did, she couldn't make her tessellation look "right."

Mr. Troy was teaching his second graders about area. To help them with the concept of covering a space, he had the students measure the area of different surfaces by covering them with sheets of scrapbook paper that were one square foot. They had already discussed the need to line up the squares so that there were no gaps or overlaps. As the students worked in groups to measure several surfaces, Mr. Troy noticed that while most groups were on their third or fourth surface, his highest ability group was still on the first one. He went over to listen to their conversation and see what was happening. While Erin sat back and watched, both Darius and Vivian were carefully aligning the squares. If they were even slightly off, they would go back and rearrange the squares. Given that the rug they were trying to measure was 32 square feet, this was quite time consuming. Every time a couple of new squares were placed, Darius or Vivian would see a square that was not precisely lined up, go readjust it, and then have to readjust every other square based on that change. Mr. Troy wondered if they would ever finish even the first part of this classroom activity.

Precision and perfection are the goals for Aggravated Accuracy Assessors. They do not take pride in the process but focus completely on the end product. Any deviation from their plan or from the "rules" creates a desperate need to repair what they are doing. They become very aggravated with themselves for not being able to do it exactly right, and they spend inordinate lengths of time redoing or refining, often at the detriment of other areas of their lives. Aggravated Accuracy Assessors often have difficulty with **goal setting**, as the only goal worthwhile in their mind is perfection, and they become so focused on creating one particular flawless work or perfecting one particular skill that they cannot divert any of their energy or attention to anything else.

Aggravated Accuracy Assessors are overly focused on precision and on a flawless final product, not enjoying or taking pride in the process.

Aggravated Accuracy Assessors are one type of unhealthy perfectionist that can result from **asynchronous development**, which is a hardship faced by many perfectionists who are gifted and talented (Morelock, 1992; Silverman, 1993a, 1993b; Tannenbaum, 1992). Gifted children's minds may develop faster than their bodies, especially when physical skills are involved, such as in art, music, and sports. Aggravated Accuracy Assessors experiencing asynchronous development often attempt the tasks but become frustrated with their inability to meet their mind's ideal. They have a perfect image in their mind and they understand the intricacies of the discipline, field, or product, yet the final product does not meet their high standards. Aggravated Accuracy Assessors constantly evaluate their products and progress and become aggravated and discouraged by their efforts and products. Often, these children will redo the same piece of work or process over and over again in an effort to make it match their mind's ideal. They may hide their works in progress, not wanting others to see their imperfect work or to offer critiques of it, and if pushed to finish a piece of work, they may frantically try to "fix" it or may just become so disappointed in their work and themselves that they give up entirely.

Perfectionism is a trait that children and adults alike exhibit in a variety of areas, not just in school. These areas can include art, music, and sports. Although a child may be a perfectionist in multiple areas, some are surprised to find that a child who is a perfectionist in one area can be so "sloppy" or not detail- or goal-oriented in another area. Several of the Aggravated Accuracy Assessors described here fall into this category. For instance, Andy's grades were falling because he was so focused on his skateboarding, and Radhika, who exhibited perfectionism in her piano playing and also in her academic achievements, did not display these same attitudes toward her softball practice or keeping her room tidy. Although Andy and Radhika both were very focused on being perfect in a particular domain and spent hours refining their skills, they did not apply this same attention to detail to other areas of their lives. In fact, they were so focused on being perfect in their chosen domain that they often did not spend the necessary time to meet others' standards in other areas. To them, nothing else mattered besides being flawless at the particular skill on which they were focused.

Perfectionism may affect a child in numerous areas of life, including academics, sports, and art. It may be focused on a specific domain or more general and pervasive.

Sometimes, Aggravated Accuracy Assessors are not focused on a particular long-term product or skill but find that their perfectionism affects many tasks at home and at school, such as Darius and Vivian trying to measure the area of a surface and Leta taking notes. Although not a project like Devon's pyramid or a skill like Andy's Ollie 540, these students were just as focused on redoing and repairing the task at hand to achieve perfection. Although the stakes may not be as high as with long-term projects, these students are just as invested in being perfect and become just as aggravated with themselves if they do not achieve perfection.

STRATEGIES FOR THE CLASSROOM

Creating high-quality products and improving a process are goals we do not want to discourage our children from, but we do want to help them use their perfectionism in a healthy manner rather than being overly aggravated with themselves, giving up on their goal, or fixating on one project. Therefore, it is essential to help Aggravated Accuracy Assessors recognize that their standards are acceptable and that they are valuable as *long-term goals*. As a teacher, you must have faith in your students' vision and their ability to meet their own expectations through *effort and revision*. This support is key for Aggravated Accuracy Assessors before you can begin helping them modify their immediate standards or goals. By reframing students' unrealistic **short-term,** or immediate, goals as **long-term goals,** you are helping them become more realistic in their expectations and more likely to experience success. Additionally, Aggravated Accuracy Assessors may need to hold conferences with you and their parents about their progress in school and at home, particularly if their focus on one goal is harming their progress in other domains.

Aggravated Accuracy Assessors have difficulty seeing the benefits of the revision process because they are so focused on the end product. They, like most students, could benefit from reading about and discussing successful people who have revised their works numerous times. You should engage students frustrated with their writing or the writing process in a discussion about the following quote by Avi, who wrote *The True Confessions of Charlotte Doyle* and *Nothing but the Truth*: "I enjoy writing, and it is hard.

> **Successful Strategies for the Classroom**
> - Recognize students' standards as acceptable as long-term goals requiring effort and revision
> - Help students reframe unrealistic short-term goals as long-term goals
> - Discuss and celebrate success as a result of revision
> - Focus on process and improvement rather than final product
> - Create a safe environment for critiquing work
> - Provide opportunities for practice and imperfection as well as to showcase final products

But then it's hard for everyone to write well. I have to rewrite over and over again so that on average it takes me a year to write a book" (Internet Public Library, 2007).

Students struggling to invent, to create, or to build something might read about Thomas Edison, who spent almost 2 years and tried more than 6,000 different carbonized plant fibers before inventing a successful light bulb, or they might read about Formula 409, which is named after the fact that the successful kitchen-cleaning formula was the 409th attempt of the two young scientists from Detroit, MI. Many students, like Ivan, struggle in art, and they would benefit from learning about examples of famous artists' works, revisions, biographies, and autobiographies that illustrate the amount of time devoted to their masterpieces. In particular, the art and life of Leonardo da Vinci's "failed" artistic experiments may show children that even famous artists do not always get it perfect. Leonardo's masterpiece, *The Last Supper*, literally began to flake off the wall even during Leonardo's lifetime due to the failed experiment of developing new types of paints. Moreover, Aggravated Accuracy Assessors who experience asynchronous development that affects their physical ability to meet their mind's ideal need to be exposed to the body of work of artists to see that skills are built over time and that success is not always immediate. It took years for Vincent van Gogh to develop his rich, expressive style and bold use of color and brushstrokes. Similarly, Pablo Picasso experimented with many different art styles before inventing Cubism. Many examples of artists' early work can be found in books, museums, and even online. Teachers can use units of study on art history or particular art movements as teachable moments for offering insight on the need for growth and improvement over time, emphasizing that many famous artists did not get their works "right" the first time.

Focusing on the process and on improvement is a way to help students not be consumed by the final product. Moreover, Aggravated Accuracy Assessors need to realize that even the "final" product can be a work in progress and that every project is an opportunity to learn and improve. You should provide your students opportunities to critique their peers' work, indicating aspects that they admire and offering constructive suggestions for improvement. You can redirect criticism of a student's work as well. For example, in looking at a student like Leta, who focuses on perfection in neatness, you could emphasize how much you like her creative ideas and encourage her to share more creativity with you. Creating a safe environment where students can discuss their works in progress and final works, whether it be writing, art, a project like Devon's pyramid, or a physical skill like piano or skateboarding, helps students begin to see what they have done successfully as well as set future goals based on what they have accomplished. As students learn to examine their own work, you should encourage them to identify not only weaknesses, which Aggravated Accuracy Assessors are used to focusing on, but also their strengths. When looking at the weaknesses, Aggravated Accuracy Assessors need guidance in setting goals to improve those weaknesses and look at them as opportunities for progress and advancement rather than as faults.

When the Aggravated Accuracy Assessors' attention to detail derails them from participating in class discussion and activities, such as with Leta who was overly focused on perfect handwriting, these students need help **prioritizing**. Especially at the elementary school level, when students are still learning and practicing their handwriting, students may not realize that there is a difference between "perfect" and "legible" or that "perfect" handwriting is not necessary in every situation. You must guide these students to help them distinguish between those times when handwriting is more important and those when it just needs to be legible. One strategy is to have students create "sloppy copies" without any erasing. You can have them write with a pen or with a pencil without an eraser. Students should write as they think, crossing or scribbling out, adding above and below lines, and drawing arrows. Some students might enjoy learning conventional editing and revising marks. This gives students permission not to assess their accuracy during the draft period, focusing more on their ideas and the content. You should take the time to call attention to your own revising process and less-than-perfect handwriting skills when jotting down ideas and notes. However, you must recognize the needs of Aggravated Accuracy Assessors to work on doing their best, including their handwriting. In addition to the "sloppy copies," students also need opportunities to use their "perfect" handwriting and to publish the work. When students are working on their final copies, you should work with them to recognize that while they will want their final copy to be neat and presentable, they do not *have to* create a perfect final piece. Help them to focus on the substance of their writing rather than just about how it looks. Some children respond well to the suggestion that irregularities in a final copy give it a personal touch. For other students, the opportunity to complete their final copy on the computer may help alleviate anxiety about making mistakes. This same process can be used for other domains, such as art. Sketching and doodling should be encouraged, as well as final products. Improvisation and sight reading may be highlighted in music lessons, along with polished compositions.

STRATEGIES FOR THE HOME

Parents of Aggravated Accuracy Assessors often become as frustrated as their children with the need for perfection. These feelings of frustration often come to a head when both parents and children are at the heights of aggravation. As a parent, you should make every effort to help your child cope with these feelings before they escalate.

One strategy is to help children set **goals** in multiple areas of their life. These goals should include not only academic goals but also social, extracurricular, and personal or self-improvement goals. The emphasis should be on a **well-balanced life** that includes many facets of a child's life. For example, in addition to improvement in spelling, a child also may add spending time playing games with friends, stop his chewing nails, and improving accuracy when shooting the basketball to his list of goals. Notice that these are **personal goals**, focused on what the child wants to improve, master, and enjoy, rather than on competitive goals like winning a competition or sport.

Successful Strategies for the Home
- Help children set goals in multiple areas of life
- Distinguish between realistic and unrealistic goals
- Distinguish between short-, medium-, and long-term goals
- Model mistakes
- Encourage children to realize their own limitations
- Discuss problems of asynchrony
- Help children prioritize

Another strategy when defining goals with children is to help them distinguish between realistic and unrealistic goals. Attaining perfection in all areas of life is an **unrealistic goal**, but improving spelling scores is a **realistic goal**. It is not realistic for a child to expect that he would not make any mistakes when recopying his class notes, but it is realistic to use a computer to help type them in a neater fashion.

Finally, goals should be classified as short-, **medium-,** or long-**term goals.** This may help children realize that while a goal may be worthwhile, it will not always happen in an immediate time frame. For example, Andy's goal of completing the skateboarding trick should have been a medium- or long-term goal. He needed time to develop his skills in other areas before he was ready to try the Ollie 540. Ivan could have developed a short-term goal to complete the Civil War drawing, while making a long-term goal to draw a portrait realistically. This may help to relieve some of the pressure that these children tend to place upon themselves.

In the discussions of goal setting, it often is important to have children recognize their own limitations. For example, a child might be able to say, "If I had all night to work on this project, I might be able to make it more perfect, but it is healthier for me to get a good night's sleep." This skill may take some time for children to develop, and parents may have to engage their children in multiple discussions before children are able to verbalize this themselves. It is important, however, for children to give themselves permission to be less than perfect.

In discussions of limitations, it may be helpful for parents to bring up issues of asynchronous development. Children may experience the frustration of the limitations from their fine motor skills or other areas of development, without the knowledge or ability to express this frustration. Explaining that a child's intellect or brain may develop faster than his or her body can catch up may help to relieve some of this anxiety.

When discussing limitations of time, it may help to have children begin to prioritize their obligations and responsibilities. Creating a **pie chart**, divided into 24 hours, may help children begin to realize how detrimental obsession in one aspect of their lives can be to other areas (see Figure 2). By realizing that when they unnecessarily spend hours on one homework activity they are missing out on other activities that they enjoy, they may be able to better prioritize their lives. Working with your child, you can help to set limits on the amount of time that should be spent on one activity, such as note taking.

When organizing how time should be spent with your child, several techniques may be helpful. A daily or weekly calendar can be a visual for students to see how they should divide their time. On the following pages, we have included a sample calendar and a blank calendar to organize children's time (see Figures 3 and 4). To keep track of the time during the afternoon or evening, many parents find the use of a kitchen timer helpful. However, for some children, this creates an additional layer of anxiety. Instead of using a timer, it may be more effective to give gentle reminders to your child, such as, "You

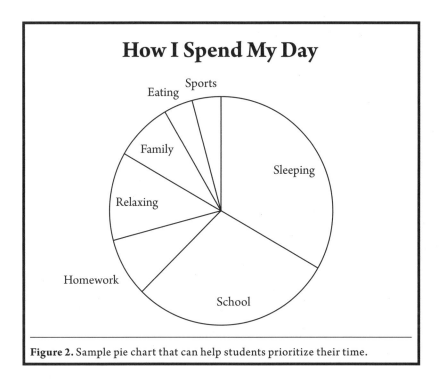

How I Spend My Day

Figure 2. Sample pie chart that can help students prioritize their time.

have about 15 more minutes to work on that," and count down at 5-minute intervals. This prepares your child to end the activity and gives him or her assistance in managing his or her time.

Finally, you can work to serve as a role model for your child's activities. You may want to point out, for example, that while having a spotless house is an important goal for you, there are still dust bunnies in the corners of the living room because it was more important to fix dinner and spend time with the family. Teachable moments in your own life may serve as excellent examples for your child's behaviors.

Although coping with an Aggravated Accuracy Assessor can be frustrating for both you and your child, strategies within the home can help to alleviate many of the stressors. You should work carefully with your child to set goals, prioritize time, and serve as a role model for managing multiple activities.

	Monday	Tuesday	Wednesday	Thursday	Friday
3:00	Snack	Snack	Snack	Snack	Snack
3:30	Homework	Homework	Homework	Homework	Project/ Study Time
4:00	Project/ Study Time	Project/ Study Time	Project/ Study Time	Project/ Study Time	Fun Reading
4:30	Flex time*	Flex time*	Flex time*	Flex time*	Flex time*
5:00	Piano Lessons	Free Time	Soccer	Free Time	Free Time
5:30	Piano Lessons	Fun Reading	Soccer	Free Time	Free Time
6:00	Dinner	Dinner	Dinner	Dinner	Dinner
6:30	Dinner/ Chores	Dinner/ Chores	Dinner/ Chores	Dinner/ Chores	Dinner/ Chores
7:00	Free Time	Family Games	Free Time	Attend Sis's Game	Friends
7:30	Free Time	Family Games	Free Time	Attend Sis's Game	Friends
8:00	Fun Reading	Family Games	Fun Reading	Fun Reading	Friends
8:30	Bedtime	Bedtime	Bedtime	Bedtime	Bedtime

Figure 3. Sample calendar.

Note. "Flex time" is to be used to finish homework, to work on ongoing projects, or to study as necessary. If all work caught up, then this is free time.

FINAL THOUGHTS

Aggravated Accuracy Assessors spend much of their time fixing their mistakes and are focused primarily on the end product. They do not understand that there are times when perfection is not expected and when being meticulous can be detrimental. The smallest per-

	Monday	Tuesday	Wednesday	Thursday	Friday
3:00					
3:30					
4:00					
4:30					
5:00					
5:30					
6:00					
6:30					
7:00					
7:30					
8:00					
8:30					

Figure 4. Blank calendar.

ceived flaw can create panic for Aggravate Accuracy Assessors, and they obsess over each little detail. Teachers and parents can help these students by emphasizing the importance of the process of getting to the end product and assisting the child in making realistic goals. This might include breaking larger long-term goals into **subtasks**, helping create timelines, discussing priorities, and providing opportunities for "sloppy copies" and for polished final copies. Examples of activities

Area of Life	Goal/ Priority	Steps to Accomplish	Check (When Completed)
Social			
Family			
Physical			
Academic			
Activities			

Figure 5. Goals worksheet.

that parents and children can complete together are shown in Figures 5 and 6. These activities can help parents and children work to develop goals and plans for meeting those goals. In subsequent chapters, you can find more resources for planning specific projects with children.

Area of Life	Specific Priority	Rank
Social		
Family		
Physical		
Academic		
Activities		
Other: _____		

Figure 6. Priorities worksheet.

5

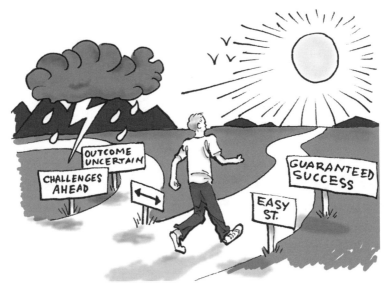

THE RISK EVADER

"All or Nothing"

Mrs. Gonzalez, the art teacher, had taught many students and was always excited when she saw an elementary student with emerging talent. One of the students with natural artistic ability was Elena. Mrs. Gonzalez had complimented her since first grade on her art-work, which consistently was above the level of detail and accuracy of her peers. Elena had a particular talent for realistic drawings, especially as her fine motor skills developed in the later elementary years. Mrs. Gonzalez had talked to Elena about her talent and had complimented her drawings in class. In fifth grade, all students were required to submit a piece of artwork for a schoolwide contest, and Elena won the overall award, receiving many accolades from the judges. However, while Elena happily drew in her notebook in the privacy of her room at home and at school during lunch and recess, she did

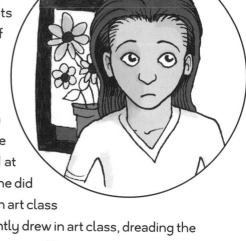

not want to participate in drawing in art class or in art competitions. She reluctantly drew in art class, dreading the appraisal that would or would not come. Despite encouragement from her parents, classroom teacher, and art teacher, she refused to enter her artwork from the schoolwide contest into the district contest. Elena did not want to risk what others would say about her artwork or that she might not win. Mrs. Gonzalez and Elena's parents lamented her decision and the missed opportunities.

Jacob really enjoyed singing and always had fun participating in the school PTA performances. He looked forward to his grade's turn to perform every year. In fourth grade, he had his heart set on a major role in the musical, which was about Lewis and Clark. His music teacher, Mrs. Lee, had commented to his mom that he had strong singing abilities for his age and should be able to earn that role. Unfortunately, Jacob became ill shortly before the try-outs, leaving him with little voice or energy on audition day. Understandably, Jacob chose not to try out that day, afraid that his illness would prevent him from performing at his best and earning him the role. His teacher talked with him and suggested he request an audition on another day, but Jacob refused to do so. Although he had told all of his friends he would earn that role, his confidence had been shaken, and he did not want to risk not being selected as the lead, even if there were other roles he also might enjoy playing.

Prairiethorpe Elementary School's academic team competed at several tournaments throughout the year. The students would study trivia and would meet for practices about twice a week. At the beginning of each semester, the coach, one of the fifth-grade teachers, would hold try-outs for the team. Lizzie's older brother had been on the team, and she had been excited about trying out since she first entered Prairiethorpe. Lizzie knew lots of trivia, and her classmates and family assumed she would get on the team. Try-out day came, and Lizzie got in line to get on the bus as usual. Her teacher knew that Lizzie would be a good addition to the team and was surprised to see her in the bus line and not headed to the try-outs. Lizzie told her that she had to go home and her mom would not let her stay. Later that month at parent-teacher conferences, Lizzie's mom commented on how disappointed Lizzie had been not to be on the academic team, and her teacher responded that it was a shame that Lizzie had to go home and miss try-outs. What they came to realize is that Lizzie had made an excuse not to try-out. When questioned about it, Lizzie finally admitted that she was afraid she wouldn't make the team and, if she did, that she wouldn't get the questions right at the tournament. Rather than take that risk, Lizzie just decided not to try out for the team.

Trey's teacher used diagnostic pretesting and **curriculum compacting**, allowing students who already mastered the content, skills, and concepts to work on **independent study projects** rather than "learning" and practicing what they already know. Trey had decided to learn about the rainforest for his independent study. He had several options for products or projects as part of his independent study, and he excitedly told his teacher he wanted to create a learning center and teach a lesson. Trey spent weeks learning all about the rainforest, focusing on the need for conservation and what people could do to help preserve the rainforest. He created activities for a learning center and was going to plan his lesson when he suddenly realized he had never taught his classmates before. They knew he was studying the rainforest, and because he was a soccer star and a good student, they were expecting to learn a lot. They talked about how fun it would be to have him as a teacher. Trey was not sure about his teaching abilities because he had not tried it before. He did not know if he would be good at it, and he was worried he would forget something or not know the answer to something. The day before he was supposed to present his lesson, Trey went to his teacher and explained that he changed his mind and did not want to teach the lesson, even though he had done all of the work and was prepared for it. He did not want to chance that he was not as prepared as he thought he was.

Kara usually sat outside at recess just watching the other girls doing cartwheels. In P.E., she would get in line at the gymnastics mats when they had centers to choose from. She would watch the other students intently, but then on her turn, she would make an excuse and move to the back of the line or another center. Kara read books about gymnastics and loved to watch it on television. When encouraged to try some gymnastics in P.E., Kara refused, and she would not join the other kids on the playground while they were doing gymnastics. One day at recess, Kara began telling her teacher all about how to do a cartwheel. Next, she started to tell her teacher about how to do flips on the bar. She could explain all of the technical aspects of the gymnastics moves and what you had to do. When her teacher found out Kara had not tried any gymnastics, even though the other kids invited her to play with them, the P.E. teacher had encouraged her, and her parents had offered to sign her up for a gymnastics class, she asked Kara why she would not try to do gymnastics. Kara explained that she knew how to do it, but she did not feel graceful and was not sure her body could do it.

Risk Evaders are afraid to take chances that might expose the fact that they are not perfect. They do not want others or themselves to see their weaknesses or to know that they are not flawless. Sometimes, especially in sports or arts requiring both mind and body, Risk Evaders may be avoiding a task due to asynchronous development, when their mind has developed faster than their body (Morelock, 1992; Silverman, 1993a, 1993b; Tannenbaum, 1992). Although they see in their mind exactly what to do and understand the skills and concepts necessary to achieve it, they are afraid that their body will not perform to their standards. They expect to be perfect the first time they try and every subsequent time. Elena could see the intricate details that a botanist sees in a flower and even could notice the pollen on the stamen, but she feared she could not produce that image present in her mature mind with her hands that had the dexterity of a 10-year-old. Although Kara could explain all of the procedural knowledge necessary to perform many gymnastics moves and even understood some of the physics behind it, she was afraid that her body could not do what her mind understood it needed to do.

It is not just asynchronous development that may cause Risk Evaders to avoid taking chances. Risk Evaders are one example of how the different descriptions of ways perfectionism is exhibited are not exclusive—for instance, Academic Achievers like Lizzie and Trey also may be Risk Evaders. The primary characteristic of Risk Evaders is that they fear failure to achieve their standards and ideals so they decide not to attempt the task. Children like Jacob might not be faced with asynchronous development or may not exhibit perfectionism in other ways, but they still are afraid that they will not meet their own expectations. They do not delight in the process or in their attempts because they are overly focused on the outcome and the possibility that it will not be perfect. Therefore, they choose not to try rather than undertake the task and possibly not succeed at a level that meets their personal standards. Risk Evaders are paralyzed by their fear, rationalizing that if they never attempt the task, they do not have to risk rejection or criticism, from themselves or from others (Adderholdt-Elliott, 1987).

STRATEGIES FOR THE CLASSROOM

As with other types of perfectionists, one of the most potent strategies for helping Risk Evaders use their perfectionism in a healthy manner is for teachers to develop a safe classroom environment that encourages risk-taking. Risk Evaders put enough pressure on themselves to be perfect and are afraid to fail without having to fear ridicule from their peers or admonishment from an authority figure. Before they will even consider taking a risk in the classroom, Risk Evaders need to feel supported within the classroom, which requires the entire class making a commitment to it being a safe environment. This environment is essential; otherwise, students fear more than just their own rejection of their work as faulty but also derision from others. To help establish a risk-taking and supportive environment, we have suggested some community-building and risk-taking activities in Chapter 9.

Risk Evaders need encouragement to try new experiences that may seem challenging and to regard these challenges as adventurous and exciting rather than as daunting. They need to be applauded for their efforts and for tackling something new instead of only being commended on their final products or successes. Without taking a risk, students cannot experience success or the delight of overcoming an obstacle. However, when they do take a risk, they need to know that the risk itself is a success because they will not be flawless or get the outcome they want every time. Helping students move their focus from being perfect to accepting challenges will give them *more* opportunities for success. Again, this all depends on the classroom being a safe environment for the students to take risks.

For some Risk Evaders, especially in the upper elementary grades, their identity may be tied to being highly successful. Thus, they may be afraid they will be seen as a fraud or imposter if they take a risk and are not flawless. Furthermore, they may have been avoiding risks for quite some time, only doing what they are certain they can succeed at. As a teacher, you need to give these students smaller opportunities for risk, although you must be careful not confuse this with opportunities for success. To be a risk, it must be a challenge to the student and the outcome must be uncertain. Although competitions are one type of risky situation that you can expose your students to, some Risk Evaders may not be ready for a statewide or districtwide competition. Instead, the classroom or even a small group of like-ability peers might provide an appropriate situation for risk-taking. You also should remember that not all risk-taking must be competitive situations, like Trey's opportunity to teach his classmates.

Some students may need even smaller opportunities for risk that can be done with minimal exposure to peers. Simply giving a piece of writing or artwork to a teacher for feedback is a big step for some students. One strategy to help students set a goal that involves a risk and then attempt it without fear of others knowing they "failed" is to have them set a goal and write it in their classroom journal or on an index card that you collect. Ask them to try something they have been afraid to try or that they have not wanted to risk. Then, have them make a plan for when and how they will try the activity. At the end of a set amount of time, have the students go back to where they wrote down the goal and reflect on the experience. Focus the children's attention on whether or not they took a risk and attempted the activity and what they gained from taking the risk rather than on whether they were successful or not. In fact, this is an excellent opportunity to help them redefine "success." If they want to share their goal and the outcome with their classmates they can and should. Otherwise, they can keep their attempt to themselves and avoid exposing the risk they took.

Risk Evaders, like Aggravated Accuracy Assessors, also need guidance in placing their focus on the process and revisions rather than only on the final outcome. By facing challenges, students can discover both their strengths and weaknesses and set future goals. Setting future goals after a risk-taking event or task sets students up to take a risk at another event or task and to focus on a specific aspect of their performance rather than only on being perfect. This also redefines success so that it is not a global evaluation of the child's performance or product compared to his or her ideal. Rather, the definition of success can be an evaluation of how he or she has progressed toward meeting his or her goals and whether he or she took a chance and tried.

STRATEGIES FOR THE HOME

One way that you, as a parent, can help Risk Evaders is to engage in family activities. These activities should be chosen to include things that all members enjoy but should not be ones that one family member is especially talented at and will dominate. Participation in these types of activities can help children realize the fun of participating in things that provide enjoyment without being skilled in them. Some example activities might include joining a community or church choir, softball league, or even informal activities, such as badminton in the backyard. Some families host karaoke nights, croquet events, or even Twister tournaments. The key is to have fun and take humor in less-than-perfect performances. Encouraging the entire family to try entirely new activities, such as whitewater rafting on vacation or dining at a new restaurant that offers unique cuisine, also can show the importance of risk-taking.

> **Successful Strategies for the Home**
> - Adopt activities that are fun but not an area of strength
> - Emphasize enjoyment over perfection
> - Upon completion of projects, notice areas of strength and improvement
> - Share joy upon completion of projects
> - Encourage intellectual risk-taking

In all activities, enjoyment should be the focus, rather than perfection. This applies to informal, extracurricular, or academic tasks. As a parent, you can help to emphasize process over product. In this way, you can help children realize the joy that comes from doing activities, rather than the frustration that comes from an emphasis on unrealistic standards.

When your child is working on a big project or assignment, you can help by taking a moment to reflect with your child when the assignment is completed. This should be done before the teacher has assessed the project. You can help your child notice his or her areas of strength in the product and also find areas for improvement. This also can be a time for celebration with your child. The key is to help your child increase **internal motivation** for completion of projects, rather than relying on the external motivation of grades and evaluations. You can help your child realize the joy that occurs when a project is completed.

This joy also can be modeled by you as a parent. When you finish a large project at work or around the house, you also can host a celebration for the family to share in the joy. These types of celebrations, even if they are as simple as ordering pizza or renting a movie at home, can provide opportunities for you and your children to discuss the joys of taking intellectual risks and finishing projects.

Finally, you can do much for your children by encouraging them to enter contests and take intellectual risks. Intellectual risks can be simple for parents to incorporate into everyday activities. For example, when selecting books, parents can encourage children to select a book a bit longer or at a slightly more advanced level. As the children are challenged by this, parents can read with their children to support their learning. Other ideas might be to watch a foreign movie with subtitles, enter a local poetry contest, or try the newspaper crossword puzzle together.

You can emphasize the benefits of trying things in which you probably will not be the winner, such as gaining experience and networking with others. Additionally, you can discuss with your children times in which you took a risk. These types of examples could include job searches or college applications. It is important to include both times in which the goal was obtained as well as others in which you were not necessarily successful. The lessons learned and benefits for this approach should be emphasized.

FINAL THOUGHTS

Risk Evaders are reluctant to try new activities or take a chance on something in which they might not be successful. This can occur in athletic, artistic, or academic domains. Sometimes, teachers and parents might perceive Risk Evaders as being lazy, as they often will choose an activity they are confident they will succeed in (usually an easier task) rather than one in which they will have to work hard to do well. However, it is these children's fear of failure and of not being perfect that is preventing them from trying more challenging activities. Teachers and parents can help Risk Evaders by developing safe environments for them to take risks and encouraging a focus on the process rather than the final outcome. They should applaud children for their efforts and for trying new, challenging activities.

6

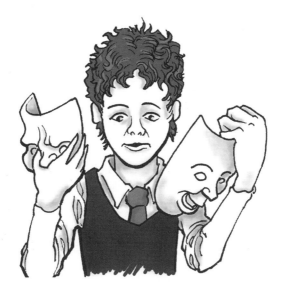

THE CONTROLLING IMAGE MANAGER

"I Could Have if I Wanted to"

Craig was somewhat athletic and loved to run and play with his friends on the playground. Recently, the majority of Craig's class has played Tag during recess. They set up boundaries that everyone had to stay within so that the arena was not too large for the size of the group. If someone stepped outside the boundaries, they automatically were "It." Craig loved to taunt whoever was It, especially when it was one of his good friends. He would run near them and yell, "You can't catch me!" However, as soon as the person who was It ran close to him, Craig would jump out of bounds, automatically making him It, declaring, "I wanted to be It!"

Rachelle was a mathematically talented fourth grader with extremely strong number sense. She was very excited when her teacher announced they would be holding a classroom tournament for Rachelle's favorite math game. Rachelle loved to play the game, and any time they had free time in the classroom she would play with her classmates or even by herself if no one else would play. When the day of the classroom tournament came, Rachelle was very focused, her skills were evident, and she easily won. Then, Rachelle competed in the schoolwide tournament, where she played the winners from the other 5 fourth-grade classes and all 6 fifth-grade classes. Rachelle again won easily against the other fourth graders and most fifth graders. In the final round, Rachelle finally was challenged somewhat, but she still won by a significant margin. Next for Rachelle was the district tournament, where the winners from all 23 elementary schools would compete. Although she was confident in her math skills, loved the game, and had been extremely successful in the classroom and schoolwide tournaments, Rachelle's teacher overhead her telling her friends that she planned to intentionally get enough penalties to disqualify her from the district tournament. When her teacher asked her about her plan, Rachelle explained that she really could win if she wanted to but she didn't want to that much. After further prompting, Rachelle admitted that math was her "thing" and she felt like she had to win but that she was not sure what her competition would be like.

Usually on report card day, Karl came home and immediately showed his mom his report card. He was an academically talented student who took pride in his grades. Plus, he knew that the local bowling alley offered 2 free games for every A and 1 free game for every B, so he loved getting to take his report card there on report card day. Karl's mom knew it was report card day, and his older brother had already given his to his mom to look at and sign. However, dinner had come and gone, and Karl still had not shown his mom his report card. She asked the boys if they were ready to go to the bowling alley, and Karl reluctantly went to get ready. Karl's mom followed him up to his room so they could talk alone, and she asked him if she could see his report card. With a great big sigh, Karl painstakingly walked over to his backpack, got out his binder, and started rummaging for his report card. Before he handed it to his mom, without looking up from his binder, he said to her, "You know, I could have gotten all A's if I wanted to. I didn't really want to this time." When she looked at Karl's report card, his mother noticed that he had earned a B+ in social studies. She asked Karl if it had been a difficult topic this marking period, and he responded, "Nah. It was just economics, but I didn't really want to get all A's. Maybe I will next time."

Latisha had been practicing and practicing her jump rope skills. No matter what her friends were playing at recess, Latisha was on the blacktop jumping rope. Sometimes she would jump rope with other children, and other times she would grab an individual rope to work on individual tricks. She had mastered many of the tricks she had seen the school's jump rope team do during their school performances. Latisha especially loved when her class was out at recess at the same time as the fourth and fifth graders because she had made a couple of friends who were on the jump rope team, and they would show her new tricks to work on. In January, the P.E. teacher held try-outs for the jump rope team, which was the first opportunity for third graders like Latisha to try out. However, Latisha decided not to go to the try-outs. The next week, when the newest members of the jump rope team were announced on the morning announcements, Latisha explained aloud that she would have made the team if she had wanted to, but she would rather just jump rope at recess instead of on a team.

Every year the PTA held an artistic competition for the elementary school students. The students submitted reflections, in the form of poetry, photography, collages, drawing, or music, on the theme for the year, which was "heroes." Mark was very excited about the competition because he had been wanting to share some of his photography. Last year, when he was in third grade, his uncle had bought him a high-tech digital camera that he had learned to use on manual mode. Mark loved his camera, and he read photography books to learn different ways of using the camera and to learn about composition. As soon as the theme for the competition was announced, Mark began thinking about what he would photograph for his submission, and he began taking even more photos than usual. When his teacher collected the submissions on the day they were due, she overheard Mark explaining to his friends that he didn't really want to win—that a "real" photographer does not need recognition and he did not submit his best photo.

Controlling Image Managers not only expect themselves to be perfect but also want others to regard them as being perfect. They do not want others to see their flaws or detect any imperfections. If they are afraid they cannot meet their own expectations or the expectations of others, they may choose to eliminate themselves intentionally to prevent failure. Rather than just choosing not to participate, as Risk Evaders will do, Controlling Image Managers set up the situation so that they can think, and say, that they *could have* succeeded and *could have been* perfect if they had *tried* or *wanted* to be successful.

Controlling Image Managers often exhibit other types of perfectionism as well. First and foremost, they often avoid risks while managing their image. Although some Controlling Image Managers, like Mark, will attempt the task but set themselves up with an explanation in the event that they do not meet expectations, other Controlling Image Managers, like Rachelle and Latisha, will avoid the task while giving an explanation that preserves their image.

> Controlling Image Managers expect themselves to be perfect and want others to see them as being perfect. Therefore, they set up situations so that they have no perceived flaws and their image as perfect is not tarnished.

Additionally, Controlling Image Managers like Karl also might be Academic Achievers. These children might have their identity so tightly connected to being academically "perfect" that they must try to control their image and identity if they exhibit anything less than academic perfection.

One problem often faced by Controlling Image Managers is that the other children they are around, such as those in their class or neighborhood, may get frustrated with them because they always must win or they "give up." For instance, the other children playing Tag with Craig never had a chance to tag him fairly. Other children may resent that Controlling Image Managers participate fully in competitive situations and only do so when they absolutely are certain they will win.

STRATEGIES FOR THE CLASSROOM

One of the important issues that must be addressed in the classroom is the frustration that other children in the class may feel because they never have a fair chance to win in a competitive situation with Controlling Image Managers. This might create tension during recess, review games in the class, and other competitive situations. One strategy to help Controlling Image Managers is to conduct some small-group role-playing, which may help Controlling Image Managers better understand others' feelings in competitive situations. Not only do they need to understand the frustration of their peers, but they also need to realize that they are

Successful Strategies for the Classroom
- Address frustrations from classmates through role-playing
- Read about and discuss role models' losses or failures and invite guest speakers to share their experiences
- Help students set personal goals, not comparative goals
- Encourage risk-taking
- Applaud student attempts and willingness to compete

not expected to be perfect or to win whenever competing against others. Controlling Image Managers would benefit from reading and discussing the losses of their role models in competitive situations. The losses might be from athletes, chess players, artists, or any other competitor, as long as they illustrate that those who chose to compete do not always win, yet are still highly regarded. Inviting guest speakers into the class to discuss their personal defeats, particularly in competitive situations, would make the idea more realistic and personal to students. They might relate to these individuals and ask these role models questions that help them come to understand the need for personal improvement and not just perfection and winning.

Unfortunately, Controlling Image Managers do not take pleasure in competition and in trying one's hardest. Instead, they focus excessively on winning and on being the best. They expect to be perfect, including being better than their classmates and friends. Controlling Image Managers need help setting personal goals that focus on their own performance prior to a competitive event, rather than focusing on how they do relative to others. This will allow them to strive for a standard that is based on their personal performance instead of relying on others being "less perfect" than them. By setting personal goals focused on their own performance, Controlling Image Managers are encouraged to compete and improve, regardless of their competition. This strategy helped Rachelle immensely. When her teacher heard her plan to eliminate herself intentionally from the district tournament, she talked with Rachelle about her personal goals for the tournament. Having personal goals that did not focus on the other students competing helped Rachelle decide to take the game home to practice and improve rather than committing to her original plan.

Like Risk Evaders, Controlling Image Managers need encouragement to try challenging, competitive situations and situations in which they are not sure they will succeed or be flawless. Again, applauding these students for their efforts and for attempting the task is essential, rather than just commending them on their final successes. Controlling Image Managers cannot truly enjoy their success or understand the feeling of accomplishment when overcoming an obstacle or winning a truly competitive situation unless they allow themselves to risk not being the best or being perfect. They must experience and come to understand that they will not always be perfect and that they will not always win but they do not have to make excuses for their performance. They need to know that they are not expected to be flawless, always to be better than others, or to never show a fault, but that they are just expected to try and to work on personal improvement.

STRATEGIES FOR THE HOME

The Controlling Image Manager can pose particular problems for parents. It can be frustrating to deal with these behaviors at home and even more difficult to help these children negotiate friendships and peer relationships. It is heartbreaking to see children lose friendships due to their own behaviors, even when parents find the same behaviors annoying.

The first step to help address this problem might be to have conversations with Controlling Image Managers during times in which they are not involved in a contest or game. When away from the controlling situation, they may be able to talk more rationally about their behavior. Additionally, it may be helpful to introduce the topic by telling the story of a similar child who does not play by

> **Successful Strategies for the Home**
> - Hold discussions during noncompetitive times
> - Role-play competitive situations
> - Play semi-competitive games at home
> - Carefully monitor competitive situations with peers or siblings and provide support
> - Find examples of competitions in media and discuss them
> - Help your child set personal goals rather than comparative goals

the rules. This may help to diffuse the situation further and allow for a deeper discussion in which your child feels less defensive. At the conclusion of the story, you then may wish to apply the lessons learned to your child's own life.

Another strategy that might be helpful is to role-play competitive situations at home. For example, you may ask your child to pretend that he or she is losing a game of checkers. Then your child could have the opportunity to react. This could be tailored to your child's interests and areas of trouble when interacting with peers. Appropriate reactions to similar situations could be the topic of a family discussion or of a conversation between you and your child. Alternatively, you could act out inappropriate reactions or play the role of your child. This may help your child to understand how his or her reactions may be frustrating to others. This type of activity should be followed with a conversation about alternative reactions that would have better outcomes. Some children might find it less threatening to talk about how someone else should react. For instance, when watching a television show or movie or reading a book and a character is losing a game, talk with your child about the different ways the character could react and how it would affect others. You might even ask your child how she or he would react if the character behaved in certain ways and they were friends. This might allow the child to see how certain behaviors are perceived by others without becoming defensive and feeling flawed.

Playing more competitive games at home also may provide opportunities to help students cope with not winning all the time. During games, whether they are sports, board games, or video games, you, as the parent, should model appropriate behavior. You also can role model good sportsmanship in accepting your wins and losses when playing games as a family. In addition, you should not allow your child to give up or get out of the situation when faced with a challenge or allow your child to succeed each time to avoid confrontation. This additional practice in authentic situations may help your child cope with his or her own imperfections. Family game time provides children with a safe environment in which to "fail."

You also have the opportunity to observe many of your child's competitive situations when he or she is interacting with peers. Formal events such as soccer games or spelling bees, as well as informal events such as play dates, provide times in which you can carefully monitor your child's interactions with peers and his or her response to competition. Prior to beginning such activities, you should plan ahead with your child to develop healthy strategies to cope with loss or even the potential for loss. These conversations can focus on helping your child set personal goals based on his or her own achievements rather than on comparing his or her performance to others. For example, the goal for a soccer game might not be to score more goals than a teammate or even to win the game. Instead, a personal goal might be to pass the soccer ball to more team members than last week. With informal events, like a play date to play board games or an outdoor game, you should talk with your child about focusing on simply having fun and enjoying the company of his or her friends rather than on always winning. You also should be aware of when your child might be exhibiting behaviors to avoid the appearance of lack of success. When these situations arise, you can be available to discuss the matter privately with your child. Finding a discreet way to make your child aware of the situation and his or her behavior may help your child to avoid such problems in the future.

Finally, it often is helpful for parents to find examples of people who have lost competitions. Examples can be found in sporting events, game shows, and even reality television shows. When a favorite team loses a game, you can emphasize that the team is still made of excellent athletes even if they lost a game. You can discuss what the team did well that day and also ask your child what the team should work on at practice before the next game. You can look at examples of Olympic athletes who did not win the gold medal, but were overjoyed to win another medal when such victory was unexpected. You can model respect for losing contestants on game shows by discussing the merits and behaviors of the players after the results are announced. The individual performance of the participants should be emphasized rather than their relative strength compared to other players.

FINAL THOUGHTS

Controlling Image Managers are especially focused on how others perceive them. They tend to set up situations so that they can think and also tell others that they *could* have succeeded if they had tried, as Craig did in the game of Tag. For them, perfection is a strong part of their identity, and they are afraid to have others see any flaws in them. Teachers and parents of Controlling Image Managers can help by encouraging risk-taking and attempts to compete. Role-playing situations also may help these children, especially if their peers are frustrated with their behavior.

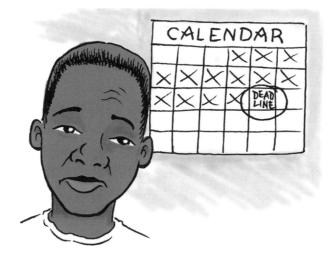

THE PROCRASTINATING PERFECTIONIST

"If It Stays in My Mind, Then I Can't Fail"

As the date for state testing neared, Elliott's teacher announced a social studies review project. The students were to create a social studies review board game over a period of several weeks. After they discussed the requirements for the project, the students went to lunch, where Elliott sat with a clipboard and began planning his game. At recess that day, Elliott excitedly shared with his teacher his intricate vision. He already had a mental picture of the board and had begun to work out the rules. Whenever his teacher or a classmate mentioned the project, Elliott got very excited and talked about his game. However, just days before the project was due, Elliott's dad asked him how the project was coming. Elliott admitted that he had not yet started on the project. Moreover, besides the plan in his head and the few sketches from that first day at lunch, Elliott did not have a plan to create his game. After a lecture from his dad, Elliott promised to work on his game, but the night before it was due, he still had not started and was not sure what to do.

Ms. Peters announced to her class that they would be competing in a national vocabulary contest. Victor was extremely excited and announced right then that he would earn a perfect score. The contest was made up of five vocabulary assessments, and students were given the vocabulary list to study prior to each assessment date. The day before the first assessment, Victor admitted to Ms. Peters that he had not yet begun studying. That night, he stayed up late studying. After he finished the contest the next day, he announced, "I didn't have enough time to study, so I couldn't get them all right."

Every night Olivia's parents struggled with her to complete her homework. She would come home from school, go to her desk, and get out her books, but by dinner she had made no progress on her homework. After dinner, she would return to her desk, but by bedtime, she still was sitting there and would break into tears because she had not completed her homework. Olivia's parents made an appointment to meet with her teacher, confused about why a young child would have so much homework. Olivia's teacher explained that the homework should only take Olivia about 30 minutes and asked about her work habits. Confused, Olivia's parents explained that she had a desk dedicated to her homework in a quiet location in the house with no television. She would sit at the desk with her homework for hours, explaining that she understood everything, but still would not complete the work by bedtime. That evening, Olivia's mom sat with her while she started on her homework. She soon realized that Olivia would sit for lengths of time staring at the paper without doing any work. She was not daydreaming or doing something else, but she just was not writing answers on the paper. When she asked Olivia what she was doing, Olivia explained that she was afraid she would write the wrong answers and would work on those problems later, and then she started looking at some other problems. This went on for the next hour, with Olivia not committing to writing any answers although she looked at every problem. When her mom asked her to tell her what she thought the answers might be, Olivia answered the majority of them correctly.

Krystal, who loved science, was very excited when her teacher passed out information about the local university's summer enrichment program. She could not believe they had a chemistry class for elementary students! Enrollment in the program was limited and thus competitive, so students were required to write an essay on why they wanted to be in the class, their parents had to complete an application form and send in a copy of the student's report card, and their teachers had to complete a recommendation form. Krystal gave the form for the recommendation to her teacher the day after she took the information home and obtained her parents' approval, and her dad copied her report card and completed the application. However, on the postmark date, Krystal still had not even begun her essay. When her dad asked her if she still wanted to go, Krystal started crying and said she wanted to go more than anything. Then when he asked her why she had not written the essay, she explained that she knew what she wanted to say but was afraid she could not write it well enough to get in. Because the deadline was fast approaching, she sat down and wrote her essay in less than 15 minutes and gave it to her dad to mail with her application.

Ryan's parents were tired of fighting with him to complete long-term projects. Every time one was assigned, they ended up helping him the night or two nights before it was due. He always had a grand vision in his mind for how to complete the project, but he never seemed to work on it before the due date was imminent. They were hoping that since Ryan now was in the fifth grade he might have matured some and learned from the stress of his previous projects. However, they found out with the first assigned project that Ryan still procrastinated when assigned a project and then panicked at the last minute. They were not sure what to do to help him. It seemed that they could not find a way to motivate him to start his project sooner.

Procrastinating Perfectionists have a perfect vision in their mind, have a perfect outcome that they expect to reach, and have very high standards for themselves and their products, but they fear that they are not able to achieve that vision. This fear paralyzes them from taking action, leading to procrastination. Unlike Risk Evaders, who intentionally do not attempt the task so that they will not fail, and unlike Controlling Image Managers, who make excuses and save face, Procrastinating Perfectionists have every intention of completing the task but just do not seem to start on it and wait until the last minute to try to accomplish it. In the back of their minds, Procrastinating Perfectionists may have thoughts that lead to inaction, such as, "If I never complete the project, I don't have to risk getting a bad grade" (Adderholdt-Elliott, 1987, p. 27) or even, "If I never complete the project, I don't have to be frustrated that the final project did not turn out the way I wanted it to or did not meet my standards."

One common incidence of procrastination for these students is long-term projects assigned at school, like those with which Elliott and Ryan struggled. When assigned a substantial project, some children, particularly gifted children, will plan elaborate and creative projects. They can see the details in their mind and become extremely enthusiastic about the project. They might share their ideas with their peers, teachers, and parents, but they are not as excited to get started on the project itself. Although they may continue to think about what they envision the final product to be like, they fear that it will not turn out the way they imagined it or are intimidated by the formidable tasks ahead and that they will not turn out perfectly. They want to do the project, but they just cannot get started on it and put it off as long as possible, until they essentially have no way of completing the project to their standards due to time constraints. Often, this leads to frustration and disappointment on their part.

Some Procrastinating Perfectionists, like Victor and Krystal, are paralyzed in a competitive situation by their fear of failure and not meeting their standards and their mind's ideal. Then, they use their procrastination as a way to control their image, to say to themselves or others that they could have done better if they had started sooner or had had more time, regardless of how much time they actually were given. Procrastinating Perfectionists typically have a vision of perfection in their mind, but their anxiety about not achieving it leads to procrastination, which then allows them to preserve their egos by giving them an "excuse" for not being perfect or achieving their standards.

For many parents, the continued pattern of procrastination from Procrastinating Perfectionists can be quite frustrating. They begin to feel that they constantly are nagging their children to get their schoolwork and other projects completed. Although their children might do high-quality work, particularly if they are an Academic Achiever as well, it is a constant struggle to get them to sit down and commit to completing work on the task until just before it is due. Worse, if the child also is a Aggravated Accuracy Assessor, the combination of waiting until the last minute to begin and then fixating on every detail may cause the child, and consequently his or her parents, extreme frustration, anxiety, and distress.

STRATEGIES FOR THE CLASSROOM

Procrastinating Perfectionists have a tendency to look at a project or task as a whole and to become overwhelmed with their vision and their fear that they cannot accomplish it perfectly. These children need help breaking down large tasks into smaller subtasks with concrete deadlines to help motivate them to complete parts prior to the main deadline. Educators who work with Procrastinating Perfectionists need to recognize their need for assistance and that they do have a vision but may not understand the steps necessary to commence work on the project and to begin to make the vision a reality. Students need to have ownership of their work, especially so that they can use their perfectionism in a healthy and beneficial manner in the future, so you should not provide them a preplanned set of smaller tasks, goals, and deadlines. Rather, you should work with students so that together they create a plan, breaking the larger task into smaller segments and setting goals along the way (see the example on the following pages). It is important for you to allow Procrastinating Perfectionists to continue to hold high standards and expectations for the final product, but by breaking it into smaller tasks and goals, Procrastinating Perfectionists now have a process to focus on and standards to meet along the way so that they do not become as overwhelmed and afraid that they cannot meet their standards. Figure 7 shows how a project might be broken down into parts. Furthermore, this helps Procrastinating Perfectionists shift their focus from the final product to the process and from the outcome to the effort that goes into the process. This will help them use their perfectionism in a healthy way and overcome their paralyzing fear.

When helping Procrastinating Perfectionists create subtasks and goals, you also need to help them learn how to develop schedules.

Successful Strategies for the Classroom

- Help students break large projects into smaller subtasks
- Help students create a schedule with "buffers"
- Help students recognize the need to prioritize and not overextend
- Focus on process and effort rather than on outcomes and final products
- Celebrate success throughout the learning process, not just at the final deadline or culminating event

Social Studies Review Game
Assigned: March 16
Due Date: April 21

Assignment: Create a review game for 2–4 players. Provide all of the necessary components (board, moving pieces, question cards, answers, rules, etc.). See your assignment sheet for the full description and for the scoring rubric. Be sure to refer to both of those documents when creating your game.

Tasks to be completed:

* Outline your game. Decide the objective (how to win), what the board should be like (you can design it like other games you have played), what happens when you get a question right or wrong, and how players will move on the board (if that is part of your game). *Suggested date: By March 20.*

* Create a plan. Once you have outlined your game, you will know what you need for a finished game. Look at the tasks below and your outline and also ask a parent to sit down with you and look at your family's calendar. Decide when you want to finish each piece. See the suggested dates below. *Due date: March 24.*

* Write questions and answers. Remember that you have to meet the requirements on the assignment sheet, with a certain number of questions per topic. When you write the questions, go ahead and record the answers. *Suggestion: Complete 3–5 questions per day.* **Due date: Have your questions written by April 14.** *Remember that Spring Break is April 4–13, so you might want to do extra at the beginning so you don't have to do as many during Spring Break!*

* Revise cards. On April 14, we will have a session to read each other's questions and make suggestions. *Suggested completion date: Have your cards revised by April 17 so your family has time to play your game and you can make further revisions, if needed, before the final due date.*

* Create your board. Your board will have to match your outline. Think about special squares, how to win, when players will answer questions, etc. This is your chance to be creative, but remember that you have a time limit and most of your points will come from the questions, not from the board design. *Suggested date: If you have plans for Spring Break, finish this by April 3. If you will be home for Spring Break and want to work on it then, plan to have it finished by April 14.*

* Write your rules. Write your rules, making sure you include everything necessary (see the assignment sheet). Be sure to ask a family member to read your rules to see if he or she understands. *Suggested date: Have these completed by April 17.* Then have your family or friends play the game. Ask them to read the rules and play while you watch. That way you can see if you forgot to write a rule, did not write a rule clearly, or need to make any other changes.

* Gather or create other necessary materials. Don't forget about any materials you need, such as moving pieces, dice, etc. *Suggested date: Gather these by April 17 so your family or friends can play.*

Figure 7. Sample task broken down.

Note. Notice the suggestion for doing a little each day (writing questions) and creating an outline/plan using the suggestions and task list as well as the family calendar.

These children, in particular, need a schedule with "**buffers**" built into them so that when something does not go as planned or does not meet their expectations and standards, they do not feel that they have failed already and that there is no need to continue. Being able to work toward their standards and goals still is important for these students, and experiencing success along the way will help them from becoming anxious and overwhelmed with fear of failure.

In addition to creating subtasks, goals, and schedules, Procrastinating Perfectionists need help prioritizing. Children who are **overextended** with afterschool activities or who are Academic Achievers who want to be perfect in all subjects may be more prone to feeling overwhelmed and become paralyzed with fear that they cannot be perfect in all of their endeavors at the same time. These children need help examining their schedule to identify when other tests and projects are due or when they have an important extracurricular event and then determine what is most important to them. If they have an elaborate project plan or challenging goal in mind, they may need help recognizing that they might not be able to put as much effort and focus into other tasks as usual. This will help them understand that they cannot be perfect and meet their high standards in all things at all times. Procrastinating Perfectionists, particularly if they are Academic Achievers or Aggravated Accuracy Assessors, need help recognizing that something has to give and that they do have limitations to what they can accomplish, especially under deadlines. Although it is important to have high standards, to set goals, and to create subtasks, these children also need to prioritize and recognize their limits. Again, you need to help these children understand that their high standards are valid and that they can excel, but also realize and acknowledge that they cannot be flawless or "the best" at everything. They may need help to see that when they have too much to accomplish, rather than feeling overwhelmed and becoming paralyzed with fear because they cannot do it all to their standards, they sometimes must adjust their expectations and sacrifice a little of one thing to excel at something else. When working with Procrastinating Perfectionists to create subtasks, goals, and a schedule, you must help them examine the entire picture and what currently requires their attention rather than just focusing on the assigned task.

For the Procrastinating Perfectionists who use their procrastination as a way to save face and control their image, addressing their fear of failure and their tendency to procrastinate will help alleviate the ego-saving behavior that they use along with procrastination. Additionally, the focus on process and effort rather than on outcomes and evaluation of the final product will help them be able to identify strengths and weaknesses rather than directing their attention toward an absolute definition of success and failure. By doing so, their identity will not be tied entirely to the outcome, so they will not need to make excuses. Rather, they can take pride in their efforts and in the process, experiencing success at what they have done along the way, including completing subtasks and meeting midpoint goals.

STRATEGIES FOR THE HOME

Parents who have experienced the "**last-minute meltdown**" when a child has not begun, much less finished, a major project the night before the due date know the difficulty that Procrastinating Perfectionists can pose to families. In the moment when the child is approaching (or experiencing) a breakdown, the important task for you is to help your child find a way to diffuse the situation and relax his or her personal standards for the project. The goal at the last minute is to finish the project while maintaining healthy sleeping habits for your child. This might mean that your child does not have the opportunity to implement all of his or her ideas, but it is important to help your child recognize his or her own limitations given the amount of time available. Alternatively, if your child cannot finish it on his or her own (without the family helping to do the work) within the remaining time while getting adequate sleep, the goal might be to help your child accept consequences for a late project. You must be sure your child knows this is not a "free pass" or another opportunity to procrastinate. You can do this by working with your child right then to create a work plan for how to accomplish the project, not to perfection, but to the degree it can be turned in, and when it will be turned in, as close to

Successful Strategies for the Home

- Help your child find ways to relax his or her standards during crunch time
- Help your child make a plan for finishing long-term assignments
- Check in regularly with your child to help maintain good work habits
- Find nonstressful times to discuss time management with your child
- Communicate regularly with your child's teachers
- Use family projects as a way to model positive behaviors

the original due date as possible. Be sure to have your child sign this as a contract with you and hold your child to it, whether the teacher will accept late work or not.

Most importantly, you, as a parent, must work with your child to prevent these situations from happening in the first place. When projects, contests, and opportunities are announced, you have the opportunity to work with your child to develop a plan to complete the objectives. These plans should set dates for specific goals and allow time for "redos," rough drafts, and revising. After the plan is in place, you should regularly check in with your child to help him or her complete his or her goals. This may need to be done daily in the beginning but may become less frequent as your child develops independence in working toward his or her goals. The following samples in Figures 8, 9, and 10 can help parents and children work together to set reasonable goals for upcoming projects.

Sometimes it may become apparent that your child does not always convey information to you about upcoming projects and

Project Name	Social Studies State Project	
Time Period	4 weeks	Due Date March 17
Tasks	1. Pick a state	
	2. Find resources	
	3. Take notes on important facts	
	4. Write an outline/organize notes	
	5. Write a "sloppy copy" of paper	
	6. Write a final copy of paper	
	7. Plan the design for the poster	
	8. Make the illustrations for the poster	
	9. Put the poster together	

Figure 8. Sample project plan.

Project Name		
Time Period		Due Date
Tasks	1.	
	2.	
	3.	
	4.	
	5.	
	6.	
	7.	
	8.	

Figure 9. Blank project planner.

	Week 1	Week 2	Week 3	Week 4
Monday	Pick a state	Finish note taking	Begin "sloppy copy"	Write final copy
Tuesday	Look online for resources	Organize notes	Work on "sloppy copy"	Finish final copy
Wednesday	Go to library for resources	Write outline	Finish "sloppy copy"	Design Poster
Thursday	Begin writing notes	Organize bibliography	Free day	Make illustrations
Friday	Free day	Free day	Free day	Free Day
Saturday	Continue writing notes	Finish up outline	Free day	Put together poster
Sunday	Continue writing notes	Finish up outline	Finish "sloppy copy"	Put together poster

Figure 10. Sample project calendar.

activities. In this case, it is imperative that you have quality communication with your child's teachers. This communication can provide information about upcoming events as well as provide feedback about your child's progress. Truly, when parents and teachers work together, children ultimately benefit. With advances in technology, such as e-mail and class Web sites, this communication has gotten easier than ever. However, do not take all responsibility off your child. Help your child see the importance of communicating with you, and be sure to ask him or her if there are any upcoming projects or tests. If your child's school or teacher does not have students use an agenda or planner to write down homework, projects, and tests, you might purchase one or just use a small notebook where your child can write down what he or she has coming up and can share with you each night.

"When parents and teachers work together, children ultimately benefit."

The best time to talk with children about procrastination is probably not when they are in the middle of a deadline crisis. Instead, you should find nonstressful times to address these issues with your child. The consequences of postponing projects and procrastination can be discussed. In addition, you can help alleviate your child's unrealistic expectations of his or her performance on projects and help your child recognize his or her own limitations in completing projects. You should emphasize to your child that all situations pose limitations for performance and that perfection is never obtainable. Providing an example of a situation in which you had to complete a project to the best of your ability under deadline might help him or her see that in the real world, perfection is not always necessary or even ideal.

Finally, families can work together to complete large-scale projects in the home, which gives an outlet for working together in a relaxed environment rather than the stress of a last-minute school project. Projects might include home improvement, such as building a deck or painting the living room; service projects, such as making a quilt for a homeless shelter or collecting cans for a soup kitchen; craft projects for gifts or decorations; or playing on an informal athletic team. Children, as well as parents, should be involved in an active role in these projects. This provides opportunities for parents to model appropriate behaviors. It also can give parents and children time to discuss the problems that are associated with perfectionism in this context. Additionally, these projects provide "teachable moments" for parents and children to share. For example, as the parent, you may wish to point out compromises that are made during the process, such as minor imperfections in the home improvement process or less elaborate plans in the service project. You should emphasize the limitations of your own skill, time available, or other circumstances that prevented you from achieving perfection in the task. Then, you could make explicit connections to projects that your child is undergoing at a similar time. Through this process, you and your children can experience the challenges, as well as the rewards, of completing a large-scale project without procrastination.

FINAL THOUGHTS

Procrastinating Perfectionists often have grand visions for projects and final products, but they delay working on those projects until there is not enough time to finish them. This often stems from a fear of creating a less-than-perfect product or performing at less than their ideal. Some Procrastinating Perfectionists use their procrastination as a way to control their image, some use it as a way to avoid taking a risk with a new idea, and others simply cannot get past the fear that they will not be able to do as well as they envision. Teachers and parents can help Procrastinating Perfectionists by guiding them in setting

realistic goals leading up to major projects and increasing communication between home and school. They must help Procrastinating
Perfectionists with planning their time, creating goals and subtasks,
and accepting responsibility.

8

IDENTIFYING HEALTHY AND UNHEALTHY PERFECTIONISM

THERE is no magic formula that will tell you if your child or student is a perfectionist and whether he or she uses his or her perfectionism in a healthy or unhealthy manner. The truth of the matter is that many children exhibit perfectionism in some contexts, but not in all situations or environments, and that they exhibit it to varying degrees. In fact, some parents and teachers find that when they meet to discuss an issue about a child's unhealthy perfectionistic behaviors the behaviors are only being exhibited in the home or at school but not both. Similarly, a child may have perfectionistic tendencies only in sports or the arts but not in academics or even in one subject but not all academic subjects. Not only do children not consistently exhibit their perfectionistic tendencies, but they also do not consistently use it in a healthy or unhealthy manner. Depending on the context, they may exhibit perfectionism in a different way, and this is affected by many factors, including:

- if they have too many commitments and are spread too thin,
- if they are in a new situation such as a self-contained gifted and talented program or being challenged in ways they have not before,

- ▸ if they are under particular stress to succeed, or
- ▸ if they have not been getting enough sleep.

Children exhibit perfectionism differently in different contexts. In fact, teachers and parents may not see the same behaviors in a child.

THE FIVE TYPES OF PERFECTIONISM

The five types of perfectionism are generalizations from what we have observed in children as teachers and a parent. Table 6 reviews the five types of perfectionists as noted in the previous chapters. These types are not exclusive categories. That is, a child may exhibit behaviors of more than one type of perfectionism. Furthermore, no child is a particular type all of the time and in all contexts. Table 6 provides a general list of behaviors that describe each type of perfectionism. These are based on our observations and are not a definitive list. Additionally, there is no set number of characteristics that do or do not define each type. That is, you should not calculate a "score" for each type to determine if a particular child could be described as that type of perfectionist or not. Instead, we hope this table will help you identify particular behaviors the child exhibits to help you identify possible strategies for helping the child use his or her perfectionism in a healthy way.

The focus should not be on labeling a child as a certain type of perfectionist, but on finding appropriate strategies to help the child use perfectionism in a healthy way.

SIGNS OF UNHEALTHY PERFECTIONISM

Used in a healthy manner, perfectionism can lead to great accomplishments and pride in one's work. However, unhealthy perfection-

Table 6
A Summary of the Characteristics of the Five Types of Perfectionists

Type of Perfectionist	Behaviors
Academic Achievers	• Identity is tied to academic achievements and performance • Is overly focused on grades • Is concerned with less than 100%, considering missing a problem or earning an A- "failure" • Fixates on extra credit for the sake of earning the points • Focuses on mistakes, which are viewed as a sign of failure and a flaw in identity • Puts forth extreme effort and agonizes over turning in perfect work • Struggles to do homework, which is viewed as an evaluation of intelligence • Expects mastery on first exposure
Aggravated Accuracy Assessors	• Goals are focused on precision and flawless work • Focuses completely on end product and not process • Deviations from his or her plan or the "rules" results in frantic "repairing" or "redos" • Becomes aggravated at self for not doing things exactly "right" • May be experiencing asynchronous development • Constantly evaluates projects and becomes frustrated with his or her work • Repeatedly redoes work • Hides work from others

Table 6, Continued

Type of Perfectionist	Behaviors
Risk Evaders	• Is afraid of taking a chance or trying something challenging because it will expose his or her imperfections • Hides weaknesses and flaws • Fear of failure results in inaction and avoiding particular tasks • Is overly focused on outcomes and the possibility of imperfection • May be experiencing asynchronous development
Controlling Image Managers	• Wants others to perceive him or her as perfect • Focuses on avoiding others' detection of his or her flaws and imperfections • Eliminates self from competitive situations rather than not succeeding as a way to avoid the risk • Manages image by saying he or she "could have" succeeded if he or she would have attempted the task • Controls image because being perfect is tied to identity • May be resented by peers for not competing in a "fair" way
Procrastinating Perfectionists	• Fears inability to achieve vision of perfection, paralyzing him or her from action • Has intentions to start but never does or puts it off until last minute • Becomes frustrated or disappointed that when he or she finally starts, the time is limited and his or her ideal cannot be reached • Sometimes controls image by explaining his or her imperfections as a lack of time for preparation or completion • May do high-quality work but struggles to commit to working on the task and beginning the work

ism can lead to tears, frustration, anxiety, distress, underachievement, and even depression. The joy of learning and trying new things is nonexistent for those experiencing unhealthy perfectionism. Again, if your child or a student in your class seems to be experiencing extreme unhealthy perfectionism or her perfectionism is affecting her eating and sleeping habits, causing her to be withdrawn, or resulting in other signs of depression, we encourage you to seek the advice of a professional, such as a counselor or psychologist.

Figure 11 provides some signs of unhealthy perfectionism that indicate that you may wish to begin conversations with the child and utilize some of the other strategies suggested in this book (see Chapters 9 and 10 in particular), as the child might need to redirect his or her perfectionism and use it in a healthier manner.

CHARACTERISTICS OF HEALTHY PERFECTIONISM

Although parents and teachers often do not think about children's perfectionism unless it is being manifested in unhealthy ways, such as stress, unhappiness, tears, procrastination, isolation, or fear, it also is important to recognize that perfectionism can be used in healthy ways, leading to high achievement, personal satisfaction, improvement, and productivity. Children who exhibit perfectionistic behaviors need to have their standards and goals validated by their teachers and parents rather than being chastised for having standards that are "too high." Having high goals and standards is healthy for children if they recognize that it takes time, effort, and revision and practice to reach their goals and that they will make mistakes along the way. By setting short-term and **intermediate goals**, children are able to maintain their high standards but work toward them at a reasonable pace. Although children should work to improve, revising their work

Signs of Unhealthy Perfectionism
The child takes no joy in the process (is only focused on outcomes).
The child avoids challenges and risks (only engages in activities in which he or she is confident he or she will succeed).
The child is fixated on redoing work because it never meets his or her own standards.
The child makes elaborate plans for an end product but has difficulty starting the product or project.
The child hides his or her mistakes.
The child cheats in order to win (in academics, sports, or games).
The child cries or becomes otherwise upset when confronted with an error.
The child makes excuses rather than admit a fault or mistake.
The child views even small mistakes as catastrophic (e.g., a potential A- is described as "failing a test").
The child is overly focused on precision.
The child constantly evaluates his- or herself.
The child becomes frustrated when something does not come easily.
Life is unbalanced because the child is overly focused on perfection in one area.
The child has strained relationships with his or her peers due to high expectations.
The child struggles in competitive situations, creating excuses or quitting if a win is not inevitable.

Figure 11. Signs of unhealthy perfectionism.

and practicing their skills, they should maintain balance, not sacrificing sleep or other healthy habits, including time for themselves and for activity and socialization. To use their perfectionism in a healthy way, children need to recognize opportunities to learn from their mistakes and must move their focus from reaching perfection to improving and reaching specific goals through effort and revision.

High standards are not necessarily unhealthy. Children need to have high standards that they work to achieve through practice and revision.

Skills for Building Healthy Perfectionism
The child sets realistic short-term, intermediate, and long-term goals.
The child has high standards for performance.
The child focuses on improvement rather than on being flawless on the first attempt.
The child is driven by intrinsic motivation.
The child focuses on effort.
The child celebrates personal successes.
The child revises and redoes work without obsessing about minor flaws.
The child learns from his or her mistakes.
The child takes risks.
The child enjoys trying new challenges.

Figure 12. Skills for building healthy perfectionism.

Learning how to transform unhealthy perfectionism into healthy perfectionism takes time and dedication. Figure 12 provides a list of skills that can help develop healthy perfectionism in children.

TOOLS TO IDENTIFY PERFECTIONISM

As described in Chapter 2, there are several formal instruments that are used in research and clinical settings to identify perfectionism in children and adults. School counselors, gifted education professionals, and trained therapists and psychologists often have access to these instruments. Also, they are available by contacting the researchers who developed the instrument. In addition to instruments that are developed specifically to identify perfectionism, many assessments of psychological distress contain measures of unhealthy perfectionism. These instruments may be used to diagnose perfectionistic tendencies that may be hindering your child's emotional well-being.

Informal assessments made through anecdotal records kept by parents and teachers may be just as useful in identifying areas where, in what situations, and how a child exhibits perfectionistic tendencies. Many parents and teachers find it helpful to keep a journal to record incidents in which a child may be exhibiting unhealthy perfectionism. This type of information can help to detect patterns of behavior and may aid adults in identifying helpful strategies for changing behavior.

FINAL THOUGHTS

Although most people tend to view perfectionism as a primarily negative trait, perfectionism can be both healthy and unhealthy. Teachers and parents can help children change unhealthy behaviors into more positive traits. Perfectionism can be identified through various formal instruments or through informal records kept by teachers or parents. These records can be used to identify patterns of behavior and possible strategies to help young perfectionists use their perfectionism in healthy ways.

9

STRATEGIES FOR THE CLASSROOM

TEACHERS play many roles and face many challenges in their classroom. Although not all of their students exhibit perfectionistic behaviors, all teachers can share stories about students they have taught who struggle with unhealthy perfectionism. Moreover, if they were to observe their students carefully throughout the day and in multiple scenarios, such as during class, at recess, and in music or art, they might see more examples of unhealthy perfectionism than they even realized. For instance, the five types of perfectionism we have defined are based on observing just one fourth-grade classroom. In this chapter, we present an overview of the strategies we presented for each type of perfectionist (see Table 7 for more detail). Then, we share general strategies to use perfectionism in a healthy way, followed by activities to use in the classroom. Although some strategies require more one-on-one or small-group work with students, perhaps during quarterly one-on-one conferences, others can be done with the entire class and would benefit all students.

Table 7
Strategies to Promote Healthy Perfectionism in the Classroom

Type of Perfectionist	Strategies to Use
Academic Achievers	• Praise for efforts and products rather than focusing praise on high grades; focus on efforts and strategies rather than on "being smart" and earning good grades • Guide students in taking pride in the process and how to use mistakes as learning experiences • Use diagnostic testing and discuss its purposes with students • Use formative assessments as an opportunity to learn from mistakes and recognize strengths (mastery) and weaknesses
Aggravated Accuracy Assessors	• Recognize students' standards as acceptable and valuable as long-term goals and have faith in their vision and ability to meet expectations through revision and effort • Help students reframe unrealistic immediate or short-term goals as medium- or long-term goals • Facilitate a discussion on balance with parents and students • Read and discuss successful people whose success has depended on revisions • Focus on process and improvement rather than the end-product • Use constructive criticism and critique as a classroom tool, including setting goals for improvement • Provide opportunities for "rough drafts" and for polished work

Risk Evaders 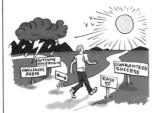	• Develop a safe classroom environment that encourages risk-taking • Encourage students to try new challenges within this safe environment • Provide opportunities for smaller risks that do not guarantee success • Applaud students for effort and trying new challenges, redefining "success" • Help students focus on process and revisions rather than final product or outcome • Have students set future goals after a risk-taking event or task
Controlling Image Managers 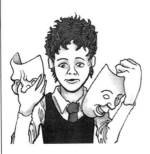	• Use small group role-playing to address social issues that arise in competitive situations at school • Read and discuss losses of role models in competitive situations • Invite guest speakers to share their personal defeats and their focus on improvement • Help students set personal goals based on their performance rather than on comparisons with peers • Encourage students and applaud them for trying challenging, competitive situations and taking risks • Applaud students for effort and risk-taking
Procrastinating Perfectionists 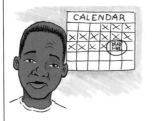	• Help students break down projects into smaller tasks and develop a schedule with "buffers" • Work with students to prioritize • Address fear of failure • Focus on process and effort rather than outcomes and products • Focus on success along the way, rather than just at the final deadline or event

GENERAL STRATEGIES TO PROMOTE HEALTHY PERFECTIONISM IN THE CLASSROOM AND TO CREATE A SUPPORTIVE ENVIRONMENT

Throughout the five chapters focusing on the different types of perfectionists, several recommendations held true for many of the types. The most important recommendation we can make for teachers is to create a safe environment for risk-taking and for learning from mistakes. Students should feel supported in the challenges they attempt and should not face ridicule from their classmates or others for trying something new. Just as you model **metacognition** and help students think about their learning, you should model risk-taking and learning from mistakes. For instance, you might share during **morning meeting** that you are taking a photography class and the challenges you are facing. (For a book on morning meetings, see Chapter 12.) You might choose to participate in a P.E., art, or music lesson, letting the students know that you are going outside your comfort zone and trying something new along with the students. When you make a mistake on the board, do not just erase it and move on. Instead, make students aware that you, like they, cannot be perfect and that mistakes do happen.

Creating an environment that is safe for risk-taking and that encourages learning from mistakes is essential for students to use their perfectionism in a healthy way.

Setting this necessary culture and climate of acceptance and safe risk-taking should begin with the first day of school. It is never too late to work with students to create this climate, but the earlier in the year it is established, the easier it is for students and you to accept it and for it to be natural. A book that we have used with children is *Be a Perfect Person in Just Three Days* by Stephen Manes. This is a great read-aloud during the first week or so of school. In the story, the main character, Milo, reads a book and fol-lows steps to become perfect in just 3 days, including wearing a stalk of broccoli around his neck for a full day. In the end, he learns that being perfect is just not fun. This can lead to immediate discussions about perfectionism and also gives a reference point for the future. When you make a mistake, you can jokingly suggest a student get a stalk of broccoli for you to wear, and similar references with students might help diffuse a situation in which they are emotionally overwhelmed by a mistake they have made or a challenge they are struggling with.

To help your class create an environment safe for risk-taking and that creates a community that works together, we recommend you spend the first couple days of school with some planned risk-taking activities and activities that are noncompetitive or cooperative. Some examples include the following:

- ► Jill took some time each day to play a class game of kickball, with the goal of supporting each other and learning the sport. By discussing the purpose and explaining that some students had never played baseball or kickball before, those who were already on baseball or softball teams naturally took on a men-toring role and would cheer for and explain the rules to their peers trying the game for the first time. Score was not the issue—learning to play as a class was the goal. (Jill purpose-fully chose teams so that they each would have a mix of nov-ices and advanced players.)
- ► A cooperative activity that gets students to interact together is the human knot. To do this, have about eight students gather in a tight circle (you will need to do multiple groups for this so that the groups are not too large). Then, have them put their right hand into the middle of the circle and hold someone else's hand (not someone immediately next to them). Next, they put in their left hand and hold another person's hand (again, not someone next to them, or the person they held

hands with before). The students then have to untangle their knot without letting go.

- ▶ Relay races and "Field Day"-type activities provide another fun opportunity for risk, especially if you do silly events that challenge the athletic students and give nonathletic students a chance so that it is a risk for everyone, and everyone can focus on having fun and working together. For instance, you could do the following activities with your class:

  - Have the students stand in a line all facing the same direction. Give the first person a ball, a roll of toilet paper, or similar object. He has to pass the object under his legs to the person behind him, who then has to pass the object over her head to the person behind her, who then passes it under his legs to the next person, and so on until it reaches the end. With toilet paper, you can have the students actually unroll it the next time and try not to break the chain. You can do this competitively (2–3 lines of students trying to do it as quickly as possible), or you can time your class and challenge them to talk together about how to improve their time before each time they repeat the activity.

  - Divide the class into several teams. Have them run a relay race with an egg on a spoon.

  - Have the students run a five-legged race (teams of four instead of partners). Then combine two groups continuously until the whole class is walking together.

  - Have the class stand in a circle holding hands. Separate two students' hands, place a hula-hoop there, and have them hold hands again. Now have the class get the hula-hoop all the way around the circle. Once they get going, add another hula-hoop and then a third. Once students have those going really well, add a hula-hoop of another color and have it go in the *opposite* direction.

► Take some time to do some creative art activities and then practice critiquing them, pointing out what students really like about them and what they think would make them more interesting. Here are some projects that are fun and relax students' standards (because art can be an area that brings out many perfectionistic tendencies):

■ Have students look at some Sumi-e painting. On her Web site (http://www.sumi-e-painting.com/sumi-e-galerie-uebersicht-gesamt.htm), Rita Böhm (n.d.) does a nice job describing the painting of flowers and birds not as copying reality but as "recreating it at [the artist's] own conception" (para. 5). This idea gives students freedom not to try to capture every detail precisely as seen. Some other aspects of the aesthetics of Japanese painting that should be discussed include simplicity of line and color and elegance of technique. To create their own paintings, first have students create a tissue paper collage background. To do this, give each student a piece of heavy white paper that is approximately 4 inches by 4 inches. Have them tear pieces of tissue paper into strips that are ½ inch to 1 inch high and 4 inches long. Mix about ⅓ water to ⅓ white glue into cups. Then have the students paint the white paper with the glue mixture and place the tissue paper strips on top. Warm colors (red, yellow, and orange) can go on the top of the paper to represent a sunset or sunrise. Cool colors (blue, violet, and green) can go on the bottom to represent the ground. It is best if the warm and cool colors do not mix. As the students lay each piece of tissue paper on the white paper, they should paint over the tissue paper with the glue mixture to secure it. The tissue paper should overlap slightly. Once those have dried, you can begin to add the Sumi-e painting on top. One non-threatening way to do this is to use straws and India ink to create a tree-like shape. India ink is inexpensive and can be found at most art supplies stores; however, black tempera paint mixed with water also will work for this project. Have the students lay their tissue paper paintings on the table on top of a larger piece of newspaper. They should move so that their face is level with the top of the table. Place a few drops of India ink on their paper and have the students blow the ink on their paper using a straw. They may want to practice this technique on some scrap paper before trying it out on their project. Let their trees dry overnight. (See Figure 13 for examples.) Once students have created their Sumi-e paintings and allowed them to dry, create a gallery, and then have students critique them. First, have them describe what is similar in all of the paintings. Then have them share what stands out in certain paintings that draw others to those particular ones. Finally, have them talk with a partner and share one thing they would do differently in their own work next time they do it. Because this is their first time critiquing, sharing with only a partner and sharing what they would change rather than what someone else would change allows students to become comfortable with this side of critiquing before having others give suggestions for improvement. As students get more involved in critiquing, you might want to use a more formal method, such as the one suggested by Joyce Payne (http://artsedge.kennedy-center. org/content/3338; to read about integrating this and other activities in language arts, see Wilson & Adelson, 2008.)

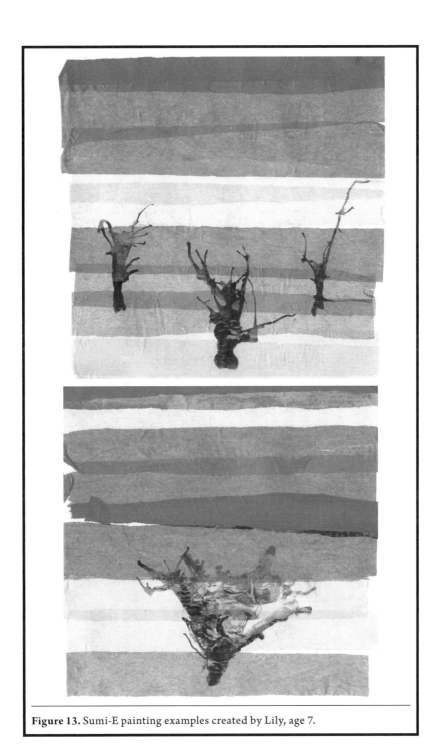

Figure 13. Sumi-E painting examples created by Lily, age 7.

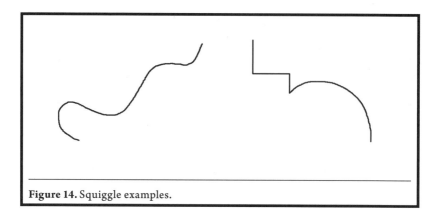

Figure 14. Squiggle examples.

- Risk-taking in school often begins with putting pencil on paper. Pass out a piece of paper with squiggles drawn on it (like the ones in Figure 14). Give students a set amount of time (2–3 minutes usually is good) to transform the squiggle into something. Have them share. Discuss which is the most original and which is the most elaborate.

▶ Give students opportunities to take academic risks as well. Provide an extension activity in mathematics, science, language arts, and social studies that will challenge them. Have each student choose one challenge to do that week. Be sure it is something that is not routine and that will challenge them. At the end of the week, have students share whether they were able to solve or complete the challenge, what they found challenging about it, and how they persisted. Be sure to define success as having tried the challenge and focus on applauding effort rather than completing or solving the challenge.

▶ Give students a colored index card. Have them write down something they have never tried before (academic, athletic, or artistic) but would like to and have the means to try in a week (cannot take months to prepare for, be too costly, involve unattainable or unavailable equipment, be out of season, etc.). Some examples might be to try in-line skating for the first time (borrowing a pair of skates from a friend), to try playing a sister's guitar, to try scrapbooking, to learn multiplication with decimals, to jump rope 200 times without missing, to write a children's picture book, to learn the capitals of all the states, to draw a self-portrait, or to conduct a particular science experiment. Post the challenges on a bulletin board and have attempting the challenges be a homework assignment due the next week—for the students to try their challenge. Again, emphasize that the goal is to *try* it. Have students report back or write a journal entry about what they tried, their emotions when trying something new, and what challenge they would like to try next.

You also might consider having a morning meeting each day. This can be just a 10–15 minute period in which you and the students greet one another and do an activity or discuss an issue together. Although we understand that time in school is stretched with many demands, this is time we have found well-spent in the classroom because it helps establish a community and helps both the teacher and students address issues in a safe place rather than having them impact the entire day. If you want more information about morning meetings, we recommend *The Morning Meeting Book* by Roxann Kriete. (See Chapter 12 for more information on this book.)

Some keys to supporting perfectionists and creating a safe environment for them to take risks and learn from mistakes is to address issues as they arrive rather than letting them build, and morning meetings gives an opportunity for this to happen. After students greet one another (perhaps by tossing a foam ball to a person while greeting him or her in a different language or by practicing "professional" handshakes to greet neighbors), you might consider allowing two or three students to share an accomplishment, helping them focus on improvement and effort, or a challenge that they faced and what happened. This would be a good time for role-playing activities as well, especially as you notice issues arising at recess, in the lunchroom, or during group work. This also might be an ideal time to have students set goals for the day, week, or marking period. At the beginning of each marking period, you might give students a colored index card and have them write three **concrete goals** focused on their own performance (not comparisons) and three steps they will take to meet those goals. These can be taped to the corner of their desk to remind them of their goals.

In general, you will want to be very aware of the language you use and the message you send to your students. Encourage students to try and to take risks, and let them know that they are not always expected to succeed on their first try. Ease students' fears before an assessment, and debrief with them after the assessment, letting them know the next steps for the class based on the results.

Most importantly, shift your focus to your students' efforts and improvements rather than just their mastery of curriculum. As teachers, we want students to master particular skills and content to be successful in life and to meet state and national standards. However, to help students reach mastery, we must focus on their efforts and improvements. This will help *all* students. For instance, our gifted and talented students often are short-changed in the current focus on standards, mastery, and meeting a level of proficiency. By focusing more on improvement, these students will continue to be challenged and learn more, even if they enter our classrooms already proficient at grade-level objectives. Moreover, as

Your words are powerful—be supportive of children and focus on their efforts, improvement, and the learning process, rather than just on outcomes and final products.

you focus on students' efforts and improvements, recognizing students for these rather than primarily for outcomes like grades, your students will take pride in their efforts and will shift their own focus to evaluating themselves on whether they have improved or not. With a focus on improvement, mastery will come! For instance, when testing students on multiplication facts, after the pretest to determine where students should start, provide students with a score indicating improvement rather than number right or wrong. So, if Joey correctly answered three more problems this time than the last time, you would write "+3" on his paper. This gives students a much more tangible, realistic short-term goal—to improve steadily—rather than an overwhelming picture of needing to master all of the facts. This also can lend itself to graphing, so that students see the upward trend as they learn more and more.

A strategy particularly useful for Procrastinating Perfectionists but one that all students would benefit from is time-management and breaking larger tasks into smaller subtasks. These are study skills that will become increasingly important as students get older and have more responsibilities. Having your students use an agenda/planner is a great method to help them take ownership for their learning, to help them make a plan for what they need to accomplish at home each evening and throughout the week, and to communicate with parents. We have seen students as young as kindergarten and first grade benefit from writing their homework in an agenda each day. If the school adopts a policy for all students to use agendas or planners (with different formats for primary and for intermediate students), students begin at an early age to develop these skills and can refine them as they get older and have more long-term projects and assignments. Be sure that students write in time to study for tests and work on projects prior to the night before the test. Personal and extracurricular goals also should be included in this process. Set goals for spending a set amount of time or studying a particular topic each night leading up to the test so that students feel prepared and do not procrastinate, staying up late the night before. In some cases, writing in free time or planned activities, such as soccer practice or piano lessons, can be helpful to students to see how they can manage their school tasks and still enjoy their other commitments or hobbies. In your morning meeting, you should address the importance of sleep and why preparing for a test or working on a project prior to the night before (or starting homework 20 minutes before bedtime) is harmful to students' future performance and learning.

ACTIVITIES TO USE IN THE CLASSROOM

Children spend many hours in school and constantly are being formally and informally evaluated by teachers, themselves, and their peers on an ongoing basis. Many types of perfectionism are exhibited within the classroom, and classroom practices can lend themselves to students exhibiting both healthy and unhealthy perfectionism. This is particularly true for children who are "schoolhouse" gifted (Renzulli, 1986) and who build their personal identity on their school accomplishments and interactions.

> Children constantly are evaluated in schools—use this as a time to help students use their perfectionism in a healthy way.

Within Existing Activities

One way that teachers can encourage healthy perfectionism rather than unhealthy perfectionism quite naturally in the classroom is through an approach that emphasizes learning from mistakes and that allows for revisions. Most teachers naturally focus on the revision process when it comes to writing, but children, particularly those in upper elementary school and middle school who receive grades on their report card, need to know that there is more to learning than getting a certain grade or percent correct. Formal assessments, including both diagnostic (or pretests) and **summative** tests (or posttests), provide an opportunity to teach children about the purposes of school and learning and to remove the focus from the final grade and perfection. This is a chance to teach children that learning is an ongoing process and that assessment is to help teachers and students determine what the students have learned and what areas they need to improve.

Diagnostic Testing (Pretesting)

Diagnostic testing is an important tool for teachers interested in differentiation, curriculum compacting, and measuring student growth. It allows the teacher and the students to determine which areas of a topic each student already has mastered, and where the child is developmentally or conceptually so that the teacher can plan learning activities accordingly. However, diagnostic tests can be a daunting task for the perfectionist, particularly the Academic Achiever. Teachers need to talk explicitly with students about the diagnostic nature of pretests, explaining what they are used for and about the expectation that students should not know everything on these tests. Encouraging students to write a question mark or "I don't know" rather than leave a question blank eases some of the pressure off them as they have *something* to write on the paper, and they know that this is acceptable.

Another useful activity with students is to give them the opportunity to compare their posttest results with their pretest results, particularly focusing on concepts that students mastered during the unit. This reframes the goal of learning from the end grade to growth and improvement, removing the pressure from achieving 100% and focusing more on progress. Teachers and parents both can help students make this transition by having them reflect on what they learned during the unit and also to set goals based on the posttest. Having children reflect on what they think they should learn or what they want to learn next, using the posttest to support their reflections, gives them the opportunity to see that continued growth and identify their own strengths and weaknesses.

Summative Assessments (Posttests)

Another way of helping children see the usefulness of assessment rather than just a final grade is to use the posttest as a learning tool. For instance, in math, after the teacher has graded students' posttests, he or she should spend a class period having students correct any problems they missed. However, teachers must keep in mind that this still has the potential to have students focus on right and wrong. One way to help them focus more on learning from their mistakes is to have them fold their paper in half vertically ("hot dog style"). The left column is labeled "Correct Answer." In this space, students show their work and find the correct answer. The right column is labeled "WIMI," which stands for "Why I Missed It." Students then explain what mistake they made. This helps students focus on concepts and process—for example, noting whether they did not understand a particular concept or whether they made a "careless" error in their arithmetic. The entire class works on helping all students master any problems that they did not answer correctly on the posttest. Students work together to teach each other missed concepts and help each other find their mistakes. When a student has corrected all of his or her missed problems and explained why he or she missed those problems, that student becomes an "expert" on the topic and is available for other students to consult with. The WIMI method works very well with mathematics because it involves concepts and process and content and skills. Students can really analyze their work and learn from the answer they originally indicated and the correct answer. This could be modified in other subject areas, depending on the type of assessment and the material assessed. Figure 15 provides an example of WIMI used with a mathematics assessment.

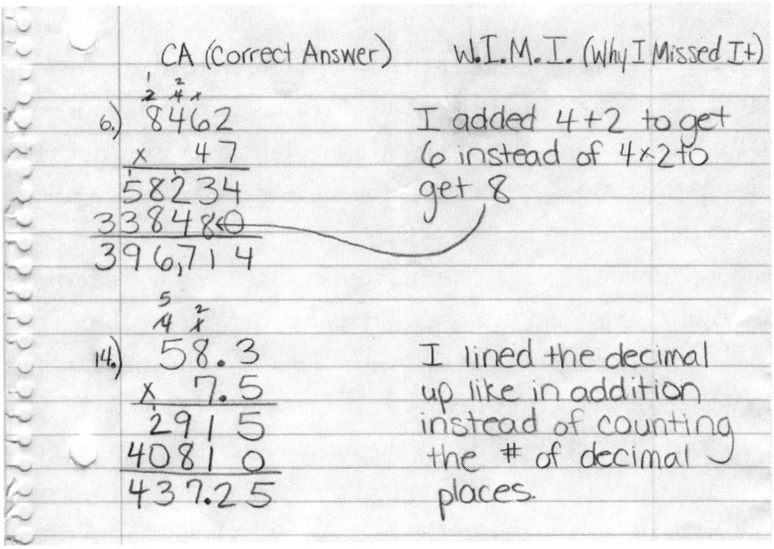

Figure 15. WIMI example.

The take-home message for teachers is to have students immediately address mistakes, misconceptions, and unlearned concepts and to learn from the posttest itself. Depending again on the topic as well as on the results, the teacher might consider creating small groups to address particular concepts or skills together, explaining how students were chosen for the group (using the data from the posttest), and then providing an opportunity for students to demonstrate their growth since the posttest through either a formal or informal assessment. Again, the teacher must explicitly have students examine their growth from the posttest to this new assessment. Otherwise, students may not realize the growth they have made and may continue to focus on the end product and their lack of perfection on the product.

Sometimes students are so focused on the final grade for a test that they lose sight of what they have learned during a particular unit of study or marking period. As mentioned before, comparing results and responses from a pretest and posttest is one strategy to help students better see what they have learned. Another strategy involves students directly reflecting on what they have learned. Before a unit, have students write in their journals, create a **mind map**, or record in another way what they already know about the topic, and collect these. At the end, have them repeat the exercise, and then pass out their original recording so that they can compare and see the growth they have made. Even just having students take a moment at the end of the test to respond to a question such as, "What are three things you learned during this unit that you did not know before?" or "What do you think you have improved on most during this unit?" (for a more skills-based unit) allows them the opportunity to reflect on their improvement and learning rather than just judge themselves by a grade. Some teachers prefer to use K-W-L (What I **K**now, What I **W**ant to Know, What I Have **L**earned) charts in their classrooms. These charts also can be used to measure what students know and learn about a topic and are easy ways for students to see how their knowledge has progressed from the beginning of the unit.

CONSTRUCTIVE CRITICISM AND FEEDBACK

Students need opportunities to reflect on their strengths and areas to improve (a more positive term than *weaknesses*) and to become comfortable with the fact that others will see high-quality aspects as well as flaws in all products that we produce. The earlier we engage students in critiquing their own work as well as the work of their peers, the more comfortable they can become with this fact and with the process of improvement. At the end of a major project or performance, have students use a rubric to reflect on how they did. This rubric could be created by the teacher, individual student, or as a whole-class activity. For primary students, rubrics can rely on visual images (i.e., smiley faces) rather than words. The resources section of this book (Chapter 12) provides several resources for teachers on the development of rubrics and Web sites with sample rubrics. On each rubric, be sure to include an open-response section in which students have to identify at least two or three strengths that they are proud of in their work as well as two or three areas that they would like to improve the next time they do a similar project (see the rubric in Figure 16). This can be related to details in the project itself, such as their attention to detail, the content knowledge that was acquired and represented, or their improvement in a particular skill, or it can be related to the process, such as their time management, their collaborative skills, or their use of the library and other resources. If you do not have time to conference with each of your students, having them do peer-critiques is an alternative way for them to discuss with someone else their strengths and the areas in which they need to improve. The "Mathematician to Mathematician" worksheet in Figure 17 is an example of how students might be guided to identify strengths and areas for improvement in their classmate's work.

ESTIMATING, HYPOTHESIZING, AND PREDICTING

As a teacher, you know these are important skills for students in many content areas, including mathematics, science, and the arts. However, these also are great opportunities to address perfectionistic tendencies with students. When students estimate, hypothesize, or predict, have them write in pen or marker so that they cannot erase what they wrote when they find out the "right answer." Talk with students about why we do these processes and about learning from them. For instance, when we "guess and test" in mathematics, our goal is to refine our "guess" each time, based on the results from when we tested the previous guess—we learn from what we did and continue. Students need to know that they are not expected to know the answer before a science experiment, before solving a mathematics problem, or before mixing colors or trying a new technique in art. We have experiences so that we can learn—if students already knew all the answers, what fun would life be? There would be no joy in learning,

Social Studies Review Game Rubric

Category	Excellent	Good	Needs Improvement	Below Expectations	Student Score	Teacher Score
Accuracy of Content	All questions and answers made for the game are correct. (up to 32 points)	All but one of the questions and answers for the game are correct. (up to 24 points)	All but two of the questions and answers for the game are correct. (up to 16 points)	Several questions and answers for the game are not accurate. (up to 8 points)		
Met Question Guidelines	Included the minimum number of questions for each category (up to 28 points)	Included the minimum number of questions for all but one category (up to 21 points)	Included the minimum number of questions for all but two categories (up to 14 points)	Did not include the minimum number of questions for more than two categories (up to 7 points)		
Rules	Rules were written clearly enough that all could easily participate. (up to 12 points)	Rules were written, but one part of the game needed slightly more explanation. (up to 9 points)	Rules were written, but people had some difficulty figuring out the game. (up to 6 points)	The rules were not written. (up to 3 points)		
Timeliness	All components submitted on time (work plan with dates, draft questions and answers, game). (up to 16 points)	One component submitted no more than 2 days late. All other components submitted on time. (up to 12 points)	Two components submitted no more than 2 days late and third component submitted on time. (up to 9 points)	A component submitted more than 2 days late, or all components late. (up to 6 points)		

Category	Excellent	Good	Needs Improvement	Below Expectations	Student Score	Teacher Score
Final Product	The board is colorful, attractive, and not messy. The questions and answers are legible. The rules are typed or written very neatly. The materials are present and stored in a convenient way. (up to 8 points)	One of the major components (board, questions and answers, rules, materials) does not meet the standards and distracts from game play. (up to 6 points)	Two of the major components (board, questions and answers, rules, materials) do not meet the standards and distract from game play. (up to 4 points)	Three of the major components (board, questions and answers, rules, materials) do not meet the standards and distract from game play. -OR- A major component interferes with the game being able to be played. (up to 2 points)		
Creativity	A lot of thought went into making the game interesting and fun to play as shown by creative questions, game pieces, and/or game board. (up to 4 points)	Some thought went into making the game interesting and fun to play by using textures, fancy writing, and/or interesting characters. (up to 3 points)	The student tried to make the game interesting and fun, but some of the things made it harder to understand/enjoy the game. (up to 2 points)	Little thought was put into making the game interesting or fun. (up to 1 point)		

Student reflection: Reflect on your project and the process of making it. On the back, write 2–3 things you did well. Then, write 2 things you could improve. These can be about a component of the game itself, your planning, or your time management.

Figure 16. Sample rubric.

Mathematician to Mathematician

(Developed by Dr. Tutita M. Casa, Project M³: Mentoring Mathematical Minds, University of Connecticut)

Please complete the following to provide feedback to your partner about her or his writing. Remember that good mathematical writing includes:

- The answers to all questions;
- Mathematical vocabulary;
- Reasons that back up the parts of your solution;
- And maybe representations (like tables, graphs, pictures, numbers, and equations).

This Stands Out!

Describe the one positive characteristic that really stood out in your partner's writing.

Words That Describe

List any vocabulary words your partner can use to make his or her thinking more clear.

Clearing Up the Mathematical Thinking

Write any questions that may help your partner make her or his response more clear. Consider starting your questions with phrases like: "Tell me more about…", "What do you mean when you say…?", "What else did you think about after you…and before you…?", and "Think about using a [representation] to show…"

Continue Doing This!

Describe any other features from your partner's writing that he or she did well.

Figure 17. Mathematician to Mathematician worksheet.

Note. Developed by Dr. Tutita M. Casa, University of Connecticut. Reprinted with permission.

Teaching process skills is an excellent opportunity to emphasize that there are moments when perfection is not expected!

and we want our students to experience that joy of discovery.

Specific Activities Addressing Perfectionism

Not only does writing naturally lend itself to opportunities to address revision and process, but it also allows an outlet for students to reflect on perfectionism and for teachers to encourage healthy expressions of perfectionism. One common pitfall of unhealthy perfectionists is that they focus on their mistakes and equate mistakes to failure. Although discussions about learning from mistakes and reading about those who have made mistakes and learned from them throughout history (such as Thomas Edison and Leonardo da Vinci) provide an intellectual understanding for perfectionists, they need to integrate this perspective of mistakes as learning experiences. One easy way to have students reflect on a healthy view of mistakes is to have them create an acrostic poem. On the left side of the paper, the student writes the letters M-I-S-T-A-K-E-S. Then, they write a word or sentence (depending on what the teacher or student chooses as the format) starting with each of those letters, focusing on how mistakes are learning opportunities. Several examples are included in Figures 18, 19, and 20.

Not only can this activity be used as a reflection piece that solidifies what a child is learning, but it also serves as a reminder to students when they do get upset about mistakes. Moreover, teachers can use this activity as a diagnostic tool, finding out how students view mistakes prior to addressing unhealthy fixation on mistakes and imperfections.

Journal writing can be cathartic for students, and it can help you identify issues that need to be addressed. You can have students write as a morning activity, a quite time after lunch before moving into the afternoon lessons, or as a means to practice their grammar and spelling.

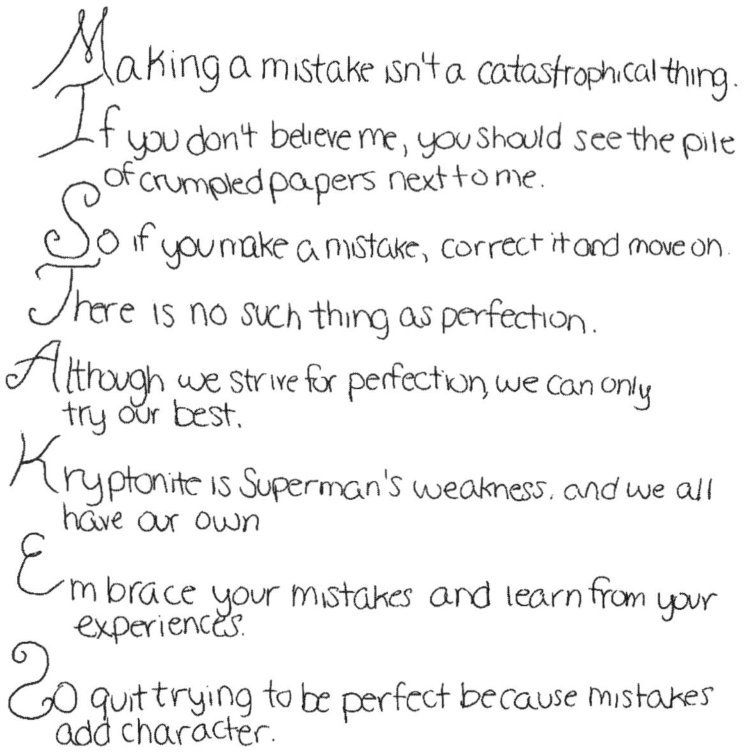

Making a mistake isn't a catastrophical thing.
If you don't believe me, you should see the pile of crumpled papers next to me.
So if you make a mistake, correct it and move on.
There is no such thing as perfection.
Although we strive for perfection, we can only try our best.
Kryptonite is Superman's weakness, and we all have our own
Embrace your mistakes and learn from your experiences.
So quit trying to be perfect because mistakes add character.

Figure 18. MISTAKE acrostic poem by Hayley of Newport News, VA.

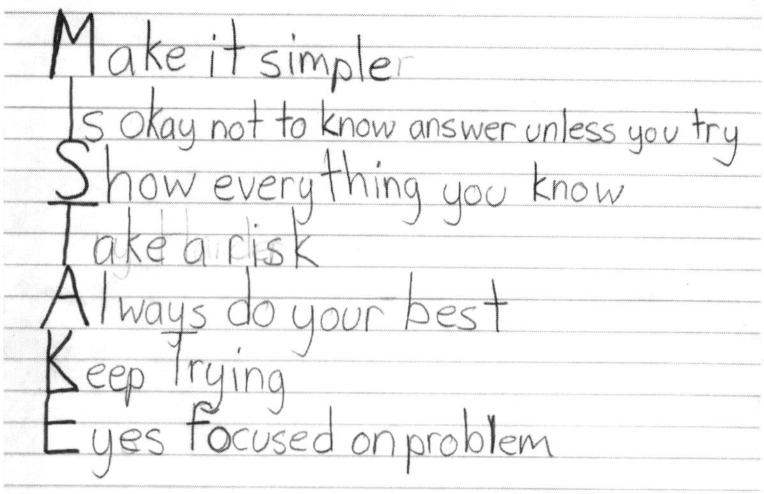

Make it simpler
Is okay not to know answer unless you try
Show everything you know
Take a risk
Always do your best
Keep Trying
Eyes focused on problem

Figure 19. MISTAKE acrostic poem by Sincham of Mansfield, CT.

Making mistakes is a great way to learn.

If you don't make mistakes, you won't learn a lot.

Stay positive and tell yourself you can do it.

Try to fix your mistake and learn from it.

m**A**kes you feel more relaxed and willing to try it again.

be **K**ind to yourself; everyone makes mistakes.

Even Albert Einstein made mistakes.

(A compilation composed from poems by Joseph, Melania, Michael, and Tim of Mansfield, CT)

Figure 20. MISTAKE acrostic poem compiled from poems by students in Mrs. Nancy Titchen's class.

Some possible journal topics include the following: responding to scenarios, setting goals and plans to reach those goals, and reflecting on how they felt before, during, and after a particular risk-taking or challenging experience. Additionally, providing quotes for students to respond to can help them think about some important issues related to perfectionism. Some quotes you might consider using include the following:

- "Forget mistakes. Forget failure. Forget everything except what you're going to do now and do it. Today is your lucky day."—Will Durant
- "If you're trying to achieve, there will be roadblocks. I've had them; everybody has had them. But obstacles don't have to stop you. If you run into a wall, don't turn around and give up. Figure out how to climb it, go through it, or work around it."—Michael Jordan
- "Fear is a part of everything you do . . . You have to take great risks to get big rewards."—Greg Louganis

- "Do one thing every day that scares you."—Eleanor Roosevelt
- "Striving for excellence motivates you; striving for perfection is demoralizing."—Harriet Braiker
- "Certain flaws are necessary for the whole. It would seem strange if old friends lacked certain quirks."—Goethe
- "No one is perfect; that is why pencils have erasers." —Unknown
- "A man would do nothing if he waited until he could do it so well that no one could find fault."—John Henry Newman

Especially as students enter the upper elementary grades, they are able to articulate their feelings. As you model learning from mistakes, taking risks, setting goals, and focusing on effort and improvement, students also take on these behaviors and develop their own strategies for using perfectionism in a healthy way. Many students are eager to share what they have learned and to help other students. Consider giving students an outlet to do this. Suggest to the art teacher that when students are learning a new technique that they be encouraged to create some art expressing a strategy they find useful when they are worried about a big project, test, or performance. Give students an opportunity to write a play or a puppet show for younger students about some of the issues you have discussed in morning meeting, such as trying a new challenge, playing fairly in games, or goal setting. Students also might enjoy writing and/or illustrating children's stories about some of these issues. You could use *Nobody's Perfect: A Story for Children About Perfectionism* by Ellen Flanagan Burns as an example. You also can have students rewrite the endings to books, stories, or biographical accounts you read, perhaps noting how the endings might have changed had everything not worked out in the protagonist's favor.

Bibliotherapy and **videotherapy** are other tools that you can use in your classroom to address perfectionism. They introduce children to characters with similar problems (Adderholdt-Elliott & Eller, 1989). According to Hébert (1991), the world of fiction, whether it be through books or movies, offers safe places for exploration, discussion, and evaluation of the behaviors of protagonists and other characters who may reflect a child's own interests, problems, and concerns. By selecting particular books and movies (see Chapter 11 for some suggestions) that feature children who exhibit perfectionistic behaviors, you provide a common situation to open a dialogue with students to address perfectionism in the classroom. By using bibliotherapy or videotherapy, you can help students identify and address issues before they become problems. In addition to stimulating discussions about issues related to perfectionism, bibliotherapy and videotherapy might make your students aware that other children have similar issues and help them identify realistic situations and articulate their own feelings. Frasier and McCannon (1981) indicated that bibliotherapy can be used in four ways in the classroom: to address an entire class problem (such as preparing for the state assessment), to address an individual problem that affects the entire class (such as Controlling Image Managers quitting during competitive situations), to address small-group problems (such as working with just Academic Achievers), and to address personal problems (such as "the development of a positive view of oneself;" p. 82). Once students have read the book or watched the video, there are many options for follow-up activities including the following:

- in-depth discussions that focus on a particular character and his or her perfectionistic behaviors;
- an art activity, such as a collage illustrating how the character was a perfectionist or a comic strip of how the character would react in a situation because he or she is a perfectionist;
- creative writing, such as writing a different resolution to a situation in which the character exhibited perfectionist tendencies or writing an internal dialogue of a character's perfectionistic thoughts;

- drama, such as role-playing, reconstructing perfectionistic behaviors with puppets, or creating and enacting a new scene with the same characters in other situations; and
- creative problem solving, graphic organizers, and other tools (be creative and let your students be creative!).

To read more about using bibliotherapy, particularly with gifted children, and for an example of using bibliotherapy to address perfectionism in high school students and in elementary and middle school students, read the article "Counseling Students Who Are Gifted Through Bibliotherapy" by Adderholdt-Elliott and Eller (1989), listed in the references and in the resources for adults (Chapter 12) or the book *Some of My Best Friends Are Books* by Judith Halsted, also listed in Chapter 12.

We know time in school is precious—integrate activities addressing perfectionism into your regular curriculum.

Take opportunities to integrate activities specifically addressing perfectionism into your regular curriculum. Just as it is good practice to integrate different content areas, students benefit greatly when you integrate aspects of social-emotional health with academic activities. For instance, when studying famous people, such as the Founding Fathers, explorers, or particular scientists, do not have students only research their contribution to history or science. Instead, also have students learn about them as people—have them research such issues as what mistakes they made and how they dealt with them and what risks they took. Not only will students be learning social-emotional skills, but this also will humanize these figures from the past, which will help students become more interested in them and retain more information about their contributions.

FINAL THOUGHTS

When addressing unhealthy perfectionism in the classroom, setting up a safe classroom environment is vital. Additionally, specific classroom activities, such as journal writing and morning meeting sessions, may help move children from unhealthy to healthy perfectionism. Teachers also have found that having students reflect on the process of creating their final products, especially through the use of rubrics, can help reduce unhealthy perfectionistic tendencies in their students.

10

STRATEGIES
FOR THE HOME

PARENTS often are perplexed by the behaviors of their children who are demonstrating perfectionistic tendencies. There are few things more frustrating to the parent of a child than the meltdowns, arguments, and anguish that can accompany perfectionism. However, there are some strategies available for parents to help their children cope and use perfectionism in a healthy way. In this chapter, we offer both advice for the "crisis moment" in which unhealthy perfectionism is rearing its ugly head as well as strategies to use in general to help children change unhealthy perfectionism into healthy perfectionism. Table 8 summarizes the strategies discussed in the previous chapters to offer help in the home for each type of perfectionist.

Throughout the previous sections, we have suggested strategies specific to each type of perfectionism. The guiding principles behind these strategies, such as discussion with children, encouraging healthy habits, and increased family activities underlie many of the examples and activities here as well. However, be sure that if you feel that your child's behavior has become unmanageable or if your child seems to be headed toward serious psychological or physical harm (such as depression, anxiety, or suicide), you pursue professional help from a psychologist, therapist, or licensed counselor. This chapter is designed to give parents who see unhealthy perfectionism in their children gen-

Table 8
Strategies to Promote Healthy Perfectionism in the Home

Type of Perfectionist	Strategies to Use
Academic Achievers	• De-emphasize grades • Celebrate learning and growth • Be an example in your mistakes • Choose books and movies to illustrate **"flawed protagonists"** • Find off-peak times to talk to your children
Aggravated Accuracy Assessors	• Help children set goals in multiple areas of life • Distinguish between realistic and unrealistic goals • Distinguish between short-, medium-, and long-term goals • Model mistakes • Encourage your children to realize their own limitations • Discuss problems of asynchrony • Help children prioritize
Risk Evaders	• Adopt activities that are fun but not an area of strength • Emphasize enjoyment over perfection • Upon completion of projects, notice areas of strength and for improvement • Share joys upon completion of projects rather than waiting for the teacher's evaluation • Encourage intellectual risk-taking
Controlling Image Managers	• Address frustrations from classmates through role-playing • Discuss competition using television, books, and other media • Help your children set personal goals, not comparative goals • Encourage risk-taking • Applaud your children's attempts and willingness to compete
Procrastinating Perfectionists	• Help your children find ways to relax standards during crunch times • Help your children make a plan for finishing long-term assignments • Check in regularly with your children to help maintain good work habits • Find nonstressful times to discuss time management with your children • Communicate regularly with your children's teachers • Use family projects as a way to model appropriate behaviors and healthy perfectionism

eral activities and strategies to guide their children toward healthier behaviors and attitudes.

"CRISIS MOMENT" STRATEGIES

Some of the most trying times as a parent can be when your child reaches what we call a "crisis moment" in his or her unhealthy perfectionism. This is the moment when a child has a meltdown or tantrum or simply shuts down. It usually is precipitated by a stressful event (i.e., a project that is due, a forthcoming competition, or a major test). At that point, the child no longer is able to function in a rational or reasonable manner, and as the parent or adult you must find a solution that will be in the best interest of the child, while acknowledging the behaviors that contributed to the crisis moment.

Of course, the best way to deal with a crisis moment is to prevent one from occurring. However, as a parent and as classroom teachers who have worked with parents and children, we know that even the best and most resourceful parents find themselves in the midst of crisis moments periodically. The general strategies in the next section of this chapter will address techniques to employ when children are more calm and able to reflect and discuss their behaviors. When your child is in the middle of a meltdown, it is not the best time to try to develop strategies that may be helpful in the future. The key to these types of situations is to neutralize the strong emotions, cope with the immediate pressures (such as due dates, competitions, and tests), and focus your child's attention to the task at hand. **Preventative measures** can be taken later.

> Your goal should be to prevent a crisis moment. However, when one occurs, you must use different strategies than you would to prevent such a moment.

When your child is in the middle of an emotional time, it is difficult for him or her to think rationally or to understand the consequences of his or her previous actions. Thus, it is important for you to help your child calm down and cope with strong emotions in order to move forward in dealing with the task at hand. As a parent, you know your child the best and what steps to take to help your child calm down. Most children are soothed through personal contact, so a hug might be the best thing for the child facing stress. Soothing music, a quiet story, a walk around the block, deep breathing, or a short nap also may be helpful. In particular, if your child has been especially stressed or has stayed up late working on a project or studying, a short nap might really help your child improve his or her state of mind and be able to deal with the situation better. Try to avoid stimulating activities, such as television, which may work to increase your child's anxiety. The important part of this stage is to bring your child to a place where he or she can begin to tackle the project.

The next step is to help your child make a plan and cope with the immediate situation. For many Procrastinating Perfectionists, it is necessary to emphasize the importance of completing a task. You should highlight the accomplishment of finishing something you have started, rather than a focus on perfection or mistakes. On a tight deadline, it may be important to ignore some details of the project in order to relieve some stress and to help your child prioritize the details that should be addressed and others that might not be as important given the time limitations. In this situation, the important thing for you is to remain calm and avoid rushing your child. Although it may be difficult given the amount of stress that you are feeling, the additional emotions inevitably will create additional stress for your child. Also, while it may be tempting to "rescue" your child by doing some of the work for him or her, this does not set your child up for future success or teach him or her how to deal with these types of moments. Working with your child to make a realistic plan and address the situation,

Resist the urge to "rescue" your child and to complete the work for him or her. Provide supports, but let your child do the work and accept the consequences for that work as well.

rather than just "solving the problem" for him or her, is important to how he or she handles future situations.

Before beginning work, take a few minutes with your child to outline a plan for completing the assignment. This may mean eliminating some of the parts of the original assignment or ideas your child has for its completion, given the time limitations. It may be helpful to have a list of "must do" and "would like to do" for the project and then decide what is realistic given the situation. This is a great tool to help your child express his or her vision for the project, yet focus on what realistically can be accomplished. Let your child know that he or she can continue to improve on a project at a later time if he or she wants, although it will be for personal satisfaction rather than for a grade or competition.

As your child begins work on the project, your role as a parent becomes crucial. It is important that your child is enabled to complete the work on his or her own. When a parent jumps in and completes the project or assignment, it reinforces the child's ideas about the need for perfection, elimination of all errors, and his or her own inadequacies. Instead, wait for your child to ask for specific help from you. Be careful to encourage your child to do tasks on his or her own, and help your child figure out ways to complete the assignment on his or her own. This will help to foster the sense of accomplishment in your child's own work. However, you should always remember that if some element of the project or product requires a potentially dangerous situation, such as hot glue, staple guns, or removing items from an oven, you should reasonably assist your child in performing these tasks (they are great moments to teach safety skills, as well!).

Throughout this process, it may become necessary to focus your child's attention to the immediate situation and work to be completed.

It is easy for children to become distracted by their emotional states, especially when they are tied to their mounting stress surrounding the project, fear of failure, and unrealistic standards. When your child begins to become worried, gently redirect his or her attention back to the project. It may be necessary to take a few moments to help him or her identify what he or she is proud about in the project. Even if your child is unable to be satisfied with the entire project, he or she should be able to identify specific areas, such as the idea or particular details. It is easy for children to waste an enormous amount of time and energy on worry and stress. You should work to create a relaxing environment for your children to work in, free from external distractions and with needed materials at hand. You may need to give your child explicit permission not to be perfect. It also is important for you to offer your unconditional love and support to your child.

GENERAL STRATEGIES

As mentioned previously, most parents would like to prevent their child from reaching the point of frustration that leads to a meltdown. Although discussing a child's unhealthy perfectionism is rarely successful during a moment of crisis, it can be quite beneficial during quiet times.

Although parents may have the tendency to lecture or address deeper issues when the child does not have control over his or her emotions, it usually is more productive to wait until times when the child is calmer, such as riding in the car or right before bed. Discussions with children about perfectionism and time management, along with purposeful family activities, can work to help change unhealthy perfectionism to healthy perfectionism.

Discussions for You and Your Child

One topic that is especially important to discuss with children is the difference between healthy and unhealthy perfectionism. A typical conversation might begin with discussing a general definition of perfectionism. This discussion should focus on specific behaviors. You and your child could identify both healthy and unhealthy behaviors. As the discussion continues about hypothetical situations, you can gently direct the conversation to situations from your child's own life. This can lead to a further discussion about healthy and unhealthy behaviors in your child's life. This might be a single discussion or a line of discussions that continues over a series of days or even weeks.

In addition, you might find teachable moments in your own life or in small examples in the life of your child to illustrate healthy or unhealthy perfectionism. Be careful about how you bring up examples of unhealthy perfectionism in your child's life. You do not want your child to feel judged or belittled. Bringing up examples in your own life and encouraging your child to think of examples from his or her life is one method of bringing these to light. If your child does not mention a particular behavior you would like to discuss, you might ask your child whether a particular behavior he or she exhibits seems unhealthy or healthy and discuss why. Remember that the purpose of the conversation is to help your child recognize these behaviors and how they help or hurt him or her, not to lecture your child or make your child feel inferior or become stressed about exhibiting perfectionistic behaviors.

Another line of discussion for parents and children is how to set goals. Goals should include not only long-term goals but also goals that could be completed in short and medium amounts of time. This might include goals for the day, week, grading period, year, and far into the future. It is important not only to emphasize the importance of goals but also to talk about the steps to take to reach the goals. For example, if one goal is to become a doctor, then learning about biology and anatomy might be short-term goals to achieve that career. Activities and behaviors should be emphasized as steps to reach the goal, rather than emphasizing outcomes, such as "making good grades." Also, keep in mind that goals should include not just academic but also social, personal, and recreational objectives. One way to help your child understand how to set short- and long-term goals is to model these as a family. Family meetings are good ways to determine a family's goal for a year, month, or week. Perhaps you set a goal as a family to travel to an amusement park for vacation over the summer. Starting in the fall, you can set the vacation as a long-term goal and then demonstrate how you can set short-term goals to achieve it, such as saving your change and counting it each week to add to a bank account for the trip. Older children can help perform certain necessary short-term tasks along the way to a long-term goal like researching options for and making airline reservations using various Internet sites. Projects around the home also are good examples of short- and long-term planning. Redecorating a child's bedroom, for instance, represents a long-term goal. Along the way, you and your child can plan short-term goals for weekend work, including trips to the hardware store for paint, priming and painting walls, or picking out new comforters or curtains. After your child understands how to apply goal setting to everyday life, use that knowledge to help him or her make goals for schoolwork or activities of interest.

Along with goal setting, parents often need to discuss with their children time management and planning for long-term projects and goals. This is particularly important for Procrastinating Perfectionists who often delay work on a project until it reaches a crisis point. It also is important for perfectionists who spend an unhealthy amount of time on a particular project or schoolwork to the neglect of friendships, family relationships, or healthy habits, such as sleep or exercise. You should help your child prioritize important parts of his or her life and organize him- or herself to spend time on each of them. In this case, it also is important for you to model these healthy habits. In modeling these habits, it may be helpful for you to look for teachable moments in the lives of famous people or characters in books, television, or movies. It is important for children to realize that even the people that they idolize make mistakes and that they have to make choices and prioritize. They also cannot excel at everything but they should try many activities. You can use moments from your own lives, admitting to your child when you make mistakes. Admitting such errors out loud and at the moment they occur can go a long way to showing your child that everyone makes mistakes in many situations.

Remember to help your child set short-, medium-, and long-term goals in academic, social, and personal areas.

Through all of these discussions, you can help your child learn how to adapt his or her unhealthy perfectionism to healthy perfectionism. You can always be on the lookout for teachable moments that might spark a conversation.

Family Time Activities

One easy way to begin family activities is to find something that family members find fun but an activity in which no one is particularly talented. This gives everyone a chance to let loose and have fun without the pressure of performing perfectly. It also will give children a safe place to fail or not to be successful. It is important in these activities that children have the chance not to be the winner in competitive situations. These activities might be physical, intellectual, or recreational, such as board games, playing Frisbee, singing karaoke, doing craft projects, or playing volleyball in the backyard.

Another family activity is to have regular celebrations of effort and process. Rather than celebrate on report card day, have a celebration at the end of the marking period *before* the report cards are sent home. This time should celebrate the hard work during the time period, rather than the child's achievement. Other examples might be to celebrate the end of a large project or the practice leading up to a big competition. These celebrations do not need to be expensive; rather, they can be simple activities. Even a trip to a favorite local restaurant, ordering pizza, having game night at home, or going to the park might be a way to celebrate a child's effort or process. Celebrating the achievement of goals for each member of the family (parents included) sets an atmosphere that treasures hard work and completion of tasks.

Many parenting resources and other experts recommend family game nights as a way for families to connect and spend time together. For families dealing with unhealthy perfectionism, game nights can serve an additional purpose. Games can provide a safe place for children to practice both winning and losing. Especially if children have trouble dealing with loss in social situations with their peer group, game nights can provide a time for children to practice losing in a supportive environment. Other families may wish to avoid competitive games and focus on games that promote cooperation, such as Family Fluxx, the Ungame, the Sleeping Grump, jigsaw puzzles, or team games. (See Chapter 11 for a description of Family Fluxx, the Ungame, and the Sleeping Grump.) These types of games can promote effort and process over achievement.

> Children often learn their values from their parents, so be sure to show them that the process and improvement made are important, not just grades and winning.

Family activities, such as game nights and celebrations of effort, can provide ways for families to enjoy each other while helping children avoid unhealthy perfectionism. Activities, along with discussion, can help parents and children work together to transition to healthy perfectionism. These activities are a starting point for families, but creative parents and children can look for other ways to connect and help combat unhealthy perfectionism.

HOMEWORK

Few parents (or children) look forward to nightly homework assignments. However, this time can be a particular struggle for families with unhealthy perfectionism. Structuring homework time to be most successful for children may help to ease the frustration and tension that often comes with it. These techniques will work for both long-term projects and short-term assignments.

The first step is to set up an environment that is conducive to studying. All children need a quiet place to complete their work, with ample space to write and adequate lighting. It also may be helpful to store school supplies and other necessities in the vicinity. It is important that this place be free from distractions such as the television and other family members playing or working. Especially for Procrastinating Perfectionists, an environment with such distractions tends to lead to many hours spent "on" homework but little of that time actually devoted to the homework. You child may enjoy and feel motivated to do projects when he or she has input into designing and setting up an ideal workspace.

In addition to creating the physical space to do homework, children also need a dedicated time each night to do homework. This need not be the exact same time each evening, as afterschool and extracurricular activities often prevent such a schedule, but you need to help your child schedule a specific time for homework each night. Write this dedicated homework time into your child's agenda or planner or on a family calendar. (For an example of planning a schedule, see the calendar in Chapter 4.)

During homework time, it is essential that you be available to support your child while he or she is working. This does not mean that you are overseeing the work or checking your child's answers. On the other hand, you should ensure that your child is able to ask you questions if he or she is unclear about an assignment or concept or to ask for help when needed. In some situations, it might be beneficial for your child to see you working on your own projects or reading a book at the same time he or she is expected to do so, setting the climate that intellectual challenges are OK and enjoyable. In other situations, this may be distracting to your child.

In addition, you should take great care not to complete your child's work for him or her or help without being asked. These behaviors can take away from your child's own sense of accomplishment in the process of completing work and emphasize the importance of the final product rather than the learning that occurs. Additionally, you should resist from always checking your child's answers (but you can check for completion when necessary). Children need to understand that homework is an opportunity to practice what they are learning and that they do not have to be perfect on each assignment. You should work with your child's teacher, finding out the homework policy, including how the teacher grades homework and whether your child receives feedback on the homework. Ideally, the focus is on practice and learning, so parents should use returned homework to talk with their child about what was learned and if further practice is needed to master the concepts.

Most children need support from their parents to plan and prioritize assignments. In less mature children, parents will need to provide more support, and as the child grows and learns he or she can build toward more independence. These are the types of life skills that you, as a parent, can help to instill in your child and that will be beneficial for your child's futures in secondary grades, college, and even the workplace. In the beginning, you may need to write a schedule with specific goals for each day with your child. Additionally, you may need to check in with your child each day to see how he or she is meeting these goals. As your child progresses, you should be able to take less of the responsibility for making the goals and check in with your child less often.

Many of the frustrations and conflicts that arise because of homework stem from miscommunication between the child and/or parent and the teacher. When parents have good communication with teachers, children benefit. At the beginning of the year, it is helpful for you, as a parent, to get information about the expectations for homework from each of your child's teachers. In particular, it is helpful to know how much time your child's teacher(s) expects him or her to spend on homework each night. If your child seems to be experiencing stress concerning assignments, then it is appropriate for you to arrange an additional meeting with your child's teacher to clear up any miscommunication. Remember that the stress may be stemming from your child's internal desires for achievement rather than from expectations from the teacher. In addition, when there is an occasion to celebrate, be sure to communicate with the teacher. It is important to convey both negative and positive events. Using a homework agenda or planner is a useful tool for communication between parents, teacher, and child. If your child's school or teacher does not require one, you might consider purchasing one for your child and teaching him or her how to use it. On this planner, the child can write upcoming projects and tests so that he or she can be preparing in advance, and parents and teacher can communicate with each other about successes or missing work.

During homework time, you can help your child by teaching him or her to accept less-than-perfect standards, especially given a reasonable amount of time. Although many children feel pressure to turn in assignments without flaws or mistakes, this expectation is unreasonable and will become increasingly difficult as the rigor of the curriculum increases. You can help your child realize the difference between ideal and reality by helping him or her to understand what expectations are realistic given the limitations of time, dexterity, and well-being. Furthermore, you should talk with your child about formative assessments, or the opportunity for him or her to practice what he or she is learning. In most cases, teachers use homework as a time for students to practice what they have learned rather than to assess mastery.

Finally, you are an important influence in your child's life when it comes to prioritizing activities. Homework and long-term projects should never compromise your child's health. For example, a regular bedtime and proper amounts of sleep are vital for your child's health and should not be extended to finish homework. At these times, you may want to consider writing a note to your child's teacher explaining the situation without necessarily asking for more time or an exception. Children do need to see that they are not expected to be perfect and sometimes we cannot fit everything into our lives but that there are consequences for the choices we make. In addition, your child may need help organizing activities, such as spending time with family and friends, as well as devoting time to school work. Healthy social relationships and a balance of fun and work are important for every person's life.

Remember that perfectionism can be used in a healthy way!

FINAL THOUGHTS

Everyone knows parenting is hard work, and parenting an unhealthy perfectionist has its own unique challenges. However, having high expectations and motivation to succeed are assets to any child. Through the strategies in this chapter, your family can build toward developing healthy behaviors and attitudes that will lead your child to greater success.

11

RESOURCES FOR CHILDREN

PICTURE BOOKS

Nobody's Perfect: A Story for Children About Perfectionism by Ellen Flanagan Burns, 2008, Magination Press

This story, written for ages 8–12, is about a young perfectionist, Sally Sanders. She worries about not measuring up and feeling like a failure. Through the sound advice of her mother and teacher, Sally learns how to overcome her perfectionism. This book provides an excellent way for children to see how their own behaviors may be connected to Sally's in the story.

Lunchtime for a Purple Snake by Harriet Ziefert, 2003, Houghton Mifflin/Walter Lorraine Books

This book describes how Jessica copes with mistakes in her artwork. Rather than starting over or throwing a fit, Jessica changes her drawings to incorporate the "mistake" into a better piece of artwork. It is a great way to teach children how mistakes can be changed into masterpieces! (Note to teachers: This is a great read-aloud for primary-aged children.)

Badly Drawn Dog by Emma Dobson, 2006, Hodder Children's Books

The protagonist in this book, a scribbly dog, goes out in search of a new identity. After much looking and shape changing, the dog realizes that his original form was the best way to be. The charming illustrations show children the benefits of being the way they are and not looking for perfection.

CHAPTER BOOKS

Be a Perfect Person in Just Three Days by Stephen Manes, 1996, Yearling Publishing

In the story, written for ages 9–12, the main character, Milo, reads a book and follows steps to become perfect in just 3 days, including wearing a stalk of broccoli around his neck for a full day. In the end, he learns that being perfect is just not fun. (Note for teachers: This is a great read-aloud during the first week or so of school.)

A Crooked Kind of Perfect by Linda Urban, 2009, Harcourt

This book, about an 11-year-old girl named Zoe, demonstrates resiliency when dreams and goals don't go as planned. Zoe, a budding musician, relies on the support of her unique family and friends and her own ingenuity to compete in a music competition. This book, filled with hope and humor, can provide role models for young perfectionists in grades 4–6.

The View from Saturday, by E. L. Konigsburg, 1998, Atheneum

Recommended for ages 9–12, this chapter book describes a sixth-grade academic trivia team. Despite the diverse group of characters, they work together to contribute to the team effort. This story of friendship can provide an excellent example of healthy competition.

The Mysterious Benedict Society, by Trenton Lee Stewart, 2008, Little, Brown and Company
Aimed at grades 5–9, this book is about a special group of gifted kids who band together to defeat the evil Mr. Curtain. Each of the characters has a unique personality and must work to overcome his or her fears throughout the adventure. This book provides role models for students to face their own fears.

Beezus and Ramona by Beverly Cleary, 1990, HarperCollins
The first in the Ramona series, this book (originally written in 1955) features Ramona's older sister, Beezus, and a preschool Ramona, who always seems to be getting into trouble. Beezus has difficulties keeping up her "perfect" persona, while less-than-perfect Ramona seems to be getting the better end of the deal. This book provides many opportunities to discuss perfectionism with children.

A Summer to Die by Lois Lowry, 2007, Delacorte Books for Young People
Meg idolizes her big sister Molly, who she sees as being absolutely perfect and flawless in every way. When Molly gets leukemia, Meg has to come to terms with both her sister's illness and her own unique gifts, in this case, photography. This book, written for a middle school audience, can provide examples of how to appreciate your gifts while accepting faults.

Rules by Cynthia Lord, 2008, Scholastic
Written for upper elementary and middle school students, this chapter book is about a girl with a brother who has autism. Through her creation of "rules" for his behavior and a developing friendship with another special needs boy, Catherine discovers deeper relationships. This book can help students redefine "normal" and develop role models.

Izzy, Willy-Nilly by Cynthia Voigt, 1986, Atheneum

Izzy has a perfect life as a cheerleader and popular student, but that is shattered when she is in a car accident that results in the loss of her leg. Throughout the book, written for middle school students, Izzy must learn to cope with her new identity and less-than-perfect life. This book can provide another role model for students who are seeking the perfect image, and learn to appreciate the inner characteristics of a person.

Millicent Min, Girl Genius by Lisa Yee, 2004, Scholastic Press

This book, written for grades 5–8, features Millie, an 11-year-old who has been accelerated into high school. Tired of being thought of as a genius, Millie uses her senior year to try to hide her abilities and have a more normal existence. However, when her new friends find out the truth, they feel betrayed and hurt. This book speaks about the importance of honesty and being true to yourself and realizing your abilities.

Stanford Wong Flunks Big-Time by Lisa Yee, 2007, Scholastic

A companion book to *Millicent Min, Girl Genius,* this book tells the story of the sixth-grade boy who Millicent tutors. Faced with enormous pressure from his family to achieve and summer school, Stanford undergoes a change of heart. Written for grades 5–8, this book can provide an example for children who feel pressure to be perfect.

(For other book suggestions, please see the Adderholdt-Elliott and Eller article listed in Chapter 12 and in the references.)

NONFICTION BOOKS

Perfectionism: What's Bad About Being Too Good **by Miriam Adderholdt and Jan Goldberg, 1999, Free Spirit**
This book, a classic in the perfectionism literature, is aimed primarily at preteen and teenage youth. Speaking directly to their audience, the authors provide advice and define terms for young perfectionists. Although some of the research that supports this book is somewhat dated, it provides valuable insights for young people.

What to Do When Good Enough Isn't Good Enough: The Real Deal on Perfectionism **by Thomas S. Greenspon, 2007, Free Spirit**
Another book speaking directly to children, it provides advice for young perfectionists. Aimed at ages 9–12, the author provides instructions for children on how to cope with perfectionism and change their negative behaviors and thought patterns.

See You Later, Procrastinator! (Get It Done) **by Pamela Espeland and Elizabeth Verdick, 2008, Free Spirit**
Part of a self-help series for kids, this illustrated nonfiction book provides tips and strategies to help kids stay on track and motivated to accomplish their goals. Using humor and full-color cartoons, this book gives procrastinators easy-to-implement strategies for changing their habits.

What to Do When You're Scared and Worried: A Guide for Kids **by James J. Crist, 2004, Free Spirit**
As part of a self-help series for kids, this book provides support for children suffering from anxiety. Dealing with both normal fears and worries and more serious problems (such as anxiety disorder and obsessive-compulsive disorder), the friendly and light tone of the book

will reassure children and give them practical strategies for coping with worries.

The Gifted Kids Survival Guide by Judy Galbraith, 2009, Free Spirit
Covering a wide variety of social and emotional issues of gifted children, this book is written directly to children ages 10 and under. It contains a chapter dealing with perfectionism and can provide support for gifted children.

The Gifted Kids Survival Guide: A Teen Handbook by Judy Galbraith and Jim Delisle, 1996, Free Spirit
Providing insights from gifted teenager's own thoughts, this book includes information about concerns faced by gifted teenagers. Including a chapter on perfectionism, this book is a great resource for older gifted students.

Smart Talk: What Kids Say About Growing Up Gifted by Robert A. Schultz and James R. Delisle, 2006, Free Spirit
This book provides stories and quotes from gifted students ages 4–12. They share their thoughts and feelings about being gifted. This book can help gifted children not feel as alone as they face the challenges of childhood.

MOVIES

Harry Potter and the Sorcerer's Stone, 2001
The popular movie about the young students at Hogwarts School of Witchcraft and Wizardry (based on the book) lends itself well to a discussion of perfectionism in the character of Hermione. Hermione, an overachieving student, can serve as an example for other children who must overcome perfectionism. One particular quote that embod-

ies Hermione's perfectionism is: "Are you sure that's a real spell? Well, it's not very good is it? I've tried a few simple spells myself, and they've all worked for me. Nobody in my family's magic at all, it was ever such a surprise when I got my letter, but I was ever so pleased, of course, it's the best school of witchcraft there is I've heard—I've learned all the course books by heart of course. I just hope it will be enough."

Harry Potter and the Prisoner of Azkaban, 2004

This is another one of the popular movies/books about Harry, Hermione, and the other students at Hogwarts School of Witchcraft and Wizardry. This one specifically provides opportunities to think about and discuss time management and the need to prioritize. Hermione, like many children with perfectionistic tendencies, has many talents and wants to succeed in them all, so she uses a Time Turner to attend extra classes that take place at the same time. This provides an opportunity to talk about limitations, scheduling, prioritizing, and decisions.

Akeelah and the Bee, 2006

Akeelah, a young girl from south Los Angeles, must overcome adversities to enter the National Spelling Bee. This movie can serve as inspiration for Risk Evaders and other children who have unhealthy perfectionism by showing them that taking intellectual risks can pay off and the benefits of perseverance. Akeelah may not always do everything perfectly, but in the end she is a winner.

WEB SITES

Gifted Kids Speak
http://www.giftedkidspeak.com
This Web site, designed for gifted children, provides stories and quotes from gifted students. Many of the concerns addressed on this Web site deal with the social and emotional issues of being gifted, including perfectionism. The forums also provide an opportunity for gifted students to participate in research projects giving voice to gifted students and the issues that surround giftedness.

Hoagies' Gifted Education: Kids and Teens
http://www.hoagiesgifted.org/hoagies_kids.htm
Part of the much larger Hoagies' Gifted Education Web site, this page provides lists and current Web sites of interest to gifted children and teenagers. It also lists books that may help gifted children relate to common social or emotional issues.

GAMES

Family Fluxx, Looney Labs
Kids may think they are about to win, when suddenly, a new card enters the picture, changing everything! In this card game, the rules constantly are being altered by the presence of new cards that can shift the game play dramatically. It's a great card game for promoting the idea of chance and the notion that sometimes going against the standard rules is really fun.

The Ungame, TaliCor
The Ungame is a noncompetitive game that fosters self-expression and communication. Expansion packs can be purchased for families,

teens, and children. As players move around the board, questions ask players to reflect on things such as, "What are the most important things in your life?" and "What do you think life will be like in 100 years?"

The Sleeping Grump, Family Pastimes

In this imaginative board game, players work together to climb the beanstalk without waking the sleeping grump. Players share their treasures and together win the game when everyone, including the grump, has his or her share. This game emphasizes cooperative work.

12

RESOURCES
FOR ADULTS

BOOKS AND ARTICLES FOR PARENTS
AND TEACHERS

"A 'Perfect' Case Study: Perfectionism in Academically Talented Fourth Graders" by Jill L. Adelson, 2007, *Gifted Child Today, 30*(4), 14–20.
The article that this book was based on, it provides case studies of perfectionism among gifted students. It provides information and background on perfectionism among elementary students.

"Counseling Students Who Are Gifted Through Bibliotherapy" by Miriam Adderholdt–Elliott and Suzanne Eller, 1989, *Teaching Exceptional Children, 22*(1), 26–31.
The authors present a rationale for using bibliotherapy, particularly with students who are gifted but also with children of all ability levels, and then explain the process of using bibliotherapy in the classroom. They provide an example using a unit on perfectionism with high school students and with elementary and middle school students. This article provides details about several fiction and nonfiction books that could be used for bibliotherapy on perfectionism, including *The Autobiography of Benjamin Franklin* by Benjamin Franklin, *Tales for*

the Perfect Child by Florence Parry Heide, *Fables* by Arnold Lobel, and *Where Do You Think You're Going, Christopher Columbus?* by Jean Fritz.

Everyone Wins: Cooperative Games and Activities by Josette Luvmour and Sambhava Luvmour, 2007, New Society Publishers
This book provides instructions for many cooperative games, appropriate for a variety of age and activity levels. These games emphasize cooperation and communication, rather than competitiveness. These games can help families and children discover the fun of participation and process, rather than a focus on the final outcome.

The Social and Emotional Development of Gifted Children: What Do We Know? edited by Maureen Neihart, Sally M. Reis, Nancy M. Robinson, and Sidney M. Moon, 2002, Prufrock Press
This comprehensive book concerning the social and emotional development of gifted children contains information on a wide variety of topics. The chapter on perfectionism provides an overview of the research concerning perfectionism in gifted children and recommendations for future research.

Some of My Best Friends Are Books: Guiding Gifted Readers From Preschool to High School by Judith Wynn Hasled, 2002, Great Potential Press
This book provides an explanation of how to use bibliotherapy with gifted children and then provides book recommendations for many of the issues that face gifted children, including perfectionism. Each list of recommendations is divided into age-appropriate selections and includes a synopsis of the book.

BOOKS FOR FAMILIES

The Good Enough Child: How to Have an Imperfect Family and Be Perfectly Satisfied by Brad E. Sachs, 2001, HarperCollins
This book provides advice for parents on how to accept your children as they come, without unrealistic expectations. The path of parenting is unpredictable, and this book provides a guide for negotiating unexpected twists and turns.

The Art of Learning: An Inner Journey to Optimal Performance by Josh Waitzkin, 2008, Free Press
The beginning of this book, written by the chess prodigy that *Searching for Bobby Fischer* was based on, describes how one family was able to allow a very talented boy avoid perfectionism and live a relatively normal childhood while still developing his talents. The insights that he provides throughout the book can serve as a model to many families in the balance of healthy and unhealthy perfectionism.

Freeing Our Families From Perfectionism by Thomas S. Greenspon, 1997, Free Spirit
Using an easy-to-read style, the author explains perfectionism and offers tips for parenting. Although the perspective includes only an unhealthy definition of perfectionism, this book provides information to help parents.

Parenting Gifted Kids: Tips for Raising Happy and Successful Children by James R. Delisle, 2006, Prufrock Press
This book provides "down-to-earth" advice for parents of gifted children. Putting forth 10 tips for parents, reflecting the author's experience with gifted children, the book focuses on changing attitudes. It includes a chapter on perfectionism, offering more tips and advice on how to help unhealthy perfectionism in children.

Raising a Gifted Child: A Parenting Success Handbook by Carol
Fertig, 2008, Prufrock Press
This easy-to-read book gives parents practical and useful advice on
parenting smart kids. It provides information on both social and emotional and academic issues facing gifted children. It empowers parents
by giving them resources to help their children.

BOOKS FOR ADULT PERFECTIONISTS

*Even June Cleaver Would Forget the Juice Box: Cut Yourself Some
Slack (and Still Raise Great Kids) in the Age of Extreme Parenting*
by Ann Dunnewold, 2007, Heath Communications
This is a fantastic book for mothers (or fathers) who are feeling the
stress and anxiety of perfectionism in their own lives. While recognizing our own shortcomings and allowing ourselves the freedom to
parent in our own styles, this book can help us to overcome perfectionism so that we can better help our children.

*When Perfect Isn't Good Enough: Strategies for Coping With Per-
fectionism* by Martin M. Anthony and Richard P. Swinson, 2009,
New Harbinger Publications
This book provides adults with strategies to overcome unhealthy perfectionism. When perfectionistic tendencies prevent you from achieving to your highest potential, this book can provide the background
information and effective strategies for coping.

*The Gifted Adult: A Revolutionary Guide for Liberating Everyday
Genius* by Mary-Elaine Jacobsen, 2000, Ballantine Books
In this book, dedicated to helping adults meet their fullest potentials,
the author provides useful advice concerning some common pitfalls
and blocks to talent development, including perfectionism. This book

is especially helpful to parents and teachers who may be trying to overcome their own sense of unhealthy perfectionism.

BOOKS FOR THE CLASSROOM

The Morning Meeting Book by Roxann Kriete, 2002, Northeast Foundation for Children
The morning meeting is a way for teachers to foster a sense of community among their students and provide time for discussing such issues as perfectionism. This book provides guidelines and examples for group activities.

BOOKS AND WEB SITES FOR CLASSROOM ASSESSMENT

Rubrics for Elementary Assessment: Classroom Ready Blackline Masters for K–6 Assessment by Nancy M. Osborne, 1998, Osborne Press
This book provides examples and masters for teachers to easily create rubrics for use in their elementary classroom. It is a great resource for teachers looking to use authentic assessment and encourage reflection in their classrooms.

Assessment: Time-Saving Procedures for Busy Teachers by Bertie Kingore, 2005, Professional Associates Publishing
This resource provides ways for teachers and students to reflect on their own work and focus on improvements and growth. It also provides templates and examples of rubrics to use with primary students, even emergent readers.

RubiStar
http://rubistar.4teachers.org
This is a free tool to help teachers create rubrics. If you register (free), you can save and edit your rubrics online and access them from school or home. This site has many templates to help you start a rubric for math, research and writing, reading, science, art, work skills, multimedia, products, music, and oral projects.

Teachnology Rubric Site
http://www.teach-nology.com/web_tools/rubrics
This site has rubric generators and makers for language arts, math, science, social studies, and more.

Rubrician
http://www.rubrician.com
This site has links to sample rubrics by category (general, language arts, math, performing arts, physical education, social studies, technology, science, and writing).

Rubrics 4 Teachers
http://www.rubrics4teachers.com
This site has links to many resources, including rubrics by subject, rubrics by term (which has many resources about rubrics), rubrics by level, and rubric tools.

Rubrics for Assessment (University of Wisconsin-Stout School of Education)
http://www.uwstout.edu/soe/profdev/rubrics.shtml
This site has links to sample rubrics as a form of online professional development. Many of these sections stand out as not being on other sites, particularly those specific to technology. Sections include quick links to rubrics; teamwork/cooperative learning rubrics; PowerPoint

and podcast rubrics; Web page and ePortfolio rubrics; video and multimedia project rubrics; virtual simulations and games rubrics; research process rubrics; writing rubrics; math, art, and science rubrics; oral presentation rubrics; rubrics for primary grades; and creating your own rubrics (templates, generators, and readings).

Kathy Schrock's Guide for Educators: Teacher Helpers: Assessment & Rubric Information

http://school.discoveryeducation.com/schrockguide/assess.html
This site has links for a lot of rubric-related resources that go beyond just rubrics. Topics include Web page rubrics, general rubrics, rubric builders, articles on rubrics, alternative assessments, electronic portfolios, graphic organizers, and report card comments.

Understanding Rubrics

http://www.middleweb.com/rubricsHG.html
This article by Heidi Goodrich Andrade includes sections on what rubrics are, why you should use them, how to create them, and what to do with them. It also includes links to samples.

Creating a Rubric: Tutorial

http://health.usf.edu/publichealth/eta/Rubric_Tutorial/default.htm
This site explains what a rubric is, why to use it, and steps to create it. At the end, it includes templates for creating your own rubrics.

TeacherVision: Creating Rubrics

http://www.teachervision.fen.com/teaching-methods-and-management/rubrics/4521.html
This site explains how one teacher designs, refines, and implements rubrics. The five parts of this tutorial address the advantages of rubrics,

creating an original rubric, analytic vs. holistic rubrics, how to weight rubrics, and student-generated rubrics.

Scholastic Professional Workshop on Rubrics: Scoring Guidelines for Performance Assessments
http://teacher.scholastic.com/professional/profdev/summerbookclubs/grade46/index.htm
This online workshop geared toward teachers in grades 4–8 includes the following sessions: introduction and examples, practice using rubrics to score student work, planning a rubric assessment for your class, and final comments with a printable certificate of completion.

BOOKS ON ANXIETY AND STRESS

Helping Your Anxious Child: A Step-by-Step Guide for Parents by Ronald M. Rapee, Ann Wignall, Susan H. Spence, Vanessa Cobham, and Heidi Lyneham, 2008, New Harbinger Publications
This book is designed for parents who have children who are experiencing extreme anxiety or have been diagnosed with anxiety disorders. It provides practical strategies and advice for parents that are based on sound research.

Anxiety-Free Kids: An Interactive Guide for Parents and Children by Bonnie Zucker, 2009, Prufrock Press
This book offers advice and strategies to help parents of children who are experiencing anxiety. It includes both a reader-friendly section for parents and a workbook for children in one volume. This guide emphasizes solutions for children and parents and involves children in the self-help process.

The Relaxation & Stress Reduction Workbook by Martha Davis, Elizabeth Robbins Eshelman, and Matthew McKay, 2008, New Harbinger Publications

This book provides instruction in the latest research-based techniques for reducing stress and anxiety among children. These powerful relaxation techniques include progressive relaxation, visualization, and mindfulness and acceptance therapy.

BOOKS ON EATING DISORDERS

Anatomy of Anorexia by Steven Levenkron, 2001, Norton

This book, written by a psychotherapist who has treated more than 300 cases of anorexia nervosa throughout his career, provides information and case studies on this disorder facing young adults. The focus of this book for parents is on early detection and it analyzes several treatment methods. This book is a valuable resource for parents who are concerned about their children and are looking for more information.

Understanding Eating Disorders: Anorexia Nervosa, Bulimia Nervosa, and Obesity edited by LeeAnn Alexander–Mott and D. Barry Lumsden, 1994, Taylor and Francis

This comprehensive book provides information about the history, treatment, and latest research pertaining to eating disorders. For parents, teachers, or other professionals looking for in-depth information concerning these three most common eating disorders, this book includes detailed background information.

WEB SITES FOR PARENTS
AND TEACHERS

Gifted Child Information Blog, Prufrock Press
http://resources.prufrock.com/GiftedChildInformationBlog/
tabid/57/Default.aspx
This blog, written by an expert in parenting gifted children, covers a
wide variety of topics relevant for parents of gifted children. She often
focuses on social and emotional issues, including perfectionism and
anxiety. She also provides links and resources that parents will find
particularly useful.

Hoagies' Gifted Education Page
http://www.hoagiesgifted.org
This site provides links for parents, educators, and kids and teens.
Along with providing general background on gifted children, it also
provides information on many social and emotional issues, including
perfectionism.

National Association for Gifted Children
http://www.nagc.org
The site for the National Association for Gifted Children provides
support for both parents and teachers of gifted children. Specific information for parents includes links to state associations that provide for
additional support for the parents of gifted children. In addition, the
site contains extensive lists of resources concerning the social and
emotional development of gifted children, including perfectionism.

The National Research Center on the Gifted and Talented (NRC/GT)
http://www.gifted.uconn.edu/NRCGT.html
This site provides research-based resources on a variety of topics in
gifted education. Many of the articles, brochures, and monographs

produced by the center are available online. Resources for parents and educators include information about social and emotional issues of gifted children, including perfectionism.

Psychology Today Perfectionism Test
http://psychologytoday.psychtests.com/tests/perfectionism_access.html
This site provides a 44-question test that takes about 20–25 minutes and addresses perfectionistic tendencies and the possible effects on your life. You get a general score describing your level of perfectionism for free, and you can also purchase scores on self-oriented, other-oriented, and social-prescribed perfectionism and advice for those types. The test was validated on a sample of 18,000.

ORGANIZATIONS

National Association for Gifted Children (NAGC)
National Association for Gifted Children
1707 L Street, N.W., Suite 550
Washington, DC 20036
Telephone: (202) 785-4268
Fax: (202) 785-4248
E-mail: nagc@nagc.org

This national organization provides support for parents, educators, and counselors of gifted children. It can provide connections to local and state organizations for additional parent support. It also publishes *Parenting for High Potential* and *Teaching for High Potential,* which often address the social and emotional issues concerning gifted children, including perfectionism.

Supporting Emotional Needs of the Gifted (SENG)
Supporting Emotional Needs of the Gifted
P.O. Box 488
Poughquag, NY 12570
Telephone: (845) 797-5054
E-mail: office@sengifted.org

This national organization is dedicated to providing resources and support to parents and educators to meet the emotional needs of the gifted. It offers a free online newsletter, resources and articles, and a directory of local parent support groups.

GLOSSARY

Academically gifted children: Children who achieve highly in academic domains or are especially talented in school-related areas, such as mathematics or verbal skills. They sometimes are referred to as "schoolhouse gifted."

Academic Achiever: One type of perfectionist who holds unrealistically high expectations for his or her performance in academic pursuits. These perfectionists focus on the final grade and on mistakes made.

Academic confidence: Belief in one's ability to do well in school and produce quality work. It sometimes referred to as "academic self-concept" or "academic self-efficacy." It is a coping resource that can help children change unhealthy perfectionism to healthy perfectionism.

Adaptive perfectionism: See Healthy perfectionism.

Aggravated Accuracy Assessor: One type of perfectionist who focuses on making every detail perfect. He or she may choose to redo the same work over and over to try to make it more like his or her mind's ideal, may look frantically for ways to "fix" the work or find the necessary materials, or may become disappointed and give up trying.

Anorexia: A serious eating disorder in which a person does not eat or eats very little. Many people suffering from anorexia display unhealthy perfectionism.

Anxiety disorders: Disabling conditions in which a person is overcome by anxiety, including stress, phobias, or fears; many people with anxiety disorders also exhibit unhealthy perfectionism.

Assessment: Any type of evaluation that a teacher, educator, or other professional might give to a student. This may include informal observations, standardized tests, or other forms of classroom grading.

Asynchronous development: A common feature of the development of children, particularly gifted children, in which one area of a child's development proceeds at a more rapid pace than another. For example, gifted children's minds may develop faster than their bodies, especially when physical skills are involved, such as in art, music, and sports.

Behavior control: How well a child is able to cooperate with others; it is a coping resource that can help children change unhealthy perfectionism to healthy perfectionism.

Bibliotherapy: A type of therapy commonly used with children, in which books are used to address common social or emotional issues.

Buffers: Time that is built into a time management plan for when something does not go as planned or does not meet expectations and standards. Buffers can help children with perfectionism because when mistakes are made, they do not feel that they have failed already and that there is no need to continue.

Bulimia: A serious eating disorder in which a person enters a cycle of binging and purging food. People suffering from bulimia often exhibit unhealthy perfectionism.

Cognitive behavior therapy: A type of therapy that focuses on adjusting the negative thought patterns, assumptions, beliefs, evaluations, and behaviors of people into more positive and healthy outcomes. This therapy has been shown to reduce unhealthy perfectionism, as well as depression and anxiety.

Concrete goals: Goals that are set by a person that have tangible and measurable outcomes. For instance, "learning five more multiplication facts this week" is a concrete goal, whereas "improving my multiplication skills" is not.

Controlling Image Manager: A type of perfectionist who wants others to regard him or her as perfect. If she is afraid she will be unable to meet her own or others' expectations in competitive situations, she may choose to eliminate herself intentionally or create a face-saving situation, saying that she *could have* been perfect.

Coping resources: An internal resource that a person can use to overcome unhealthy perfectionism. These include social confidence, behavior control, academic confidence, peer acceptance, and family support.

Creativity tests: Tests commonly used in the identification of gifted students to measure a person's creativity or divergent thinking skills. One common creativity test is the Torrance Test of Divergent Thinking.

Crisis moments: The period when unhealthy perfectionism is most difficult for parents, children, and teachers to cope. It often occurs when a child is throwing a tantrum, has completely shut down, or is overwhelmed by the current task.

Curriculum compacting: A technique commonly used with advanced learners, in which teachers give a diagnostic assessment to assess what portions of an upcoming unit of study a student has already mastered and then replace material the student already has mastered with a more appropriate learning activity.

Depression: A serious condition in which a person feels sad or down for an extended period of time and that interferes with daily life and normal functioning or causes pain. Unhealthy perfectionism often is associated with depression.

Diagnostic assessment or test: A type of assessment used at the beginning of a course of study to document the level of mastery a student has achieved prior to beginning instruction. This also is referred to as preassessment or pretesting.

Dichotomous thinking: The tendency to view events in life as either bad or good, with little or no "gray area" in between. This type of thinking often is associated with unhealthy perfectionism.

Eating disorders: Serious conditions in which a person persists in unhealthy eating habits, such as anorexia or bulimia. People with eating disorders often exhibit unhealthy perfectionism.

Extrinsic rewards: Rewards for achievement that exist outside of a person, for example, praise from a teacher, stickers, or candy.

Family support: The degree of support from family; it is a coping resource that can help children change unhealthy perfectionism to healthy perfectionism.

Fear of failure: One sign of unhealthy perfectionism; an intense fear of failure can prevent some people from trying new activities, taking risks, or attempting challenges.

Flawed protagonist: The lead character in a story, movie, or book who makes mistakes, has character defects, or displays imperfections in other ways.

Formal assessments: Evaluations given by teachers, educators, or other professionals that document learning or mastery. Formal assessments tend to be written, such as a standardized test or a unit test developed by the teacher. They also may take the form of a rubric to document more subjective evaluations.

Formative assessments: These are assessments that typically are given at the beginning or during of a unit of study to evaluate student mastery of concepts, skills, or knowledge so that the educator can assess students' current knowledge and skills and plan further instruction and learning experiences. Diagnostic assessments are one type of formative assessment.

Gifted children: According to the 1988 federal definition, children and youth who give evidence of high performance capability in areas such as *intellectual, creative, artistic,* or *leadership* capacity, or in *specific academic fields,* and who require services or activities not ordinarily provided by the school in order to fully develop such capabilities.

Goal setting: The process of making goals and developing a plan for reaching those goals. This is a common way to help unhealthy perfectionists develop healthier habits.

Goals: Objectives that one sets in hopes of reaching them within a set period of time.

Healthy perfectionism: Sometimes called normal or adaptive perfectionism; represents the characteristics that are positive for students, including gaining a sense of pride from achievements and improvement and a drive for success.

Imposter syndrome: Common to some types of unhealthy perfectionism, it occurs when a person believes that other people's confidence in him or her is unwarranted. Those who experience imposter syndrome often have an intense fear of failure and need to mask their mistakes for fear of "discovery."

Independent study projects: One way that teachers adapt the curriculum for advanced learners; students are allowed to study a topic of their own interest and develop a project to demonstrate their learning. Teachers may choose to have students create and sign a contract describing the work they will do and how it will be assessed or evaluated.

Informal assessments: Evaluations that rely primarily on observation and less documented forms of evidence of student mastery or growth. Common informal assessments include anecdotal records, mind maps, or discussions with students.

Instruments: Tests, assessments, or evaluation procedures that are used to diagnose, evaluate, or document various psychological constructs.

Intermediate goals: Goals that are set for an intermediate amount of time, usually between a few weeks and a few months. These also are referred to as medium-term goals.

Internal motivation: Motivation to accomplish tasks that come from inside of a person; for example, internal motivation often comes from a "drive to succeed" or a "love of learning."

Intrinsic motivation: See Internal motivation.

Intrinsic rewards: Rewards that come from within a person. For example, it often is described as the "joy of discovery" when learning a new concept.

Last-minute meltdown: When a child has not begun, much less finished, a major project the night before, or very close to, the due date and panics. This often occurs with Procrastinating Perfectionists.

Learning goals: Measurable goals for a student's learning, or mastery of content within the school curriculum.

Long-term goals: Goals that are set for a longer period of time, typically between 1 and 5 years.

Maladaptive perfectionism: See Unhealthy perfectionism.

Medium-term goal: See Intermediate goal.

Metacognition: A tool for teaching in which students are instructed to think or reflect on their own thinking processes.

Mind map: A type of graphic organizer that allows students to record and organize their knowledge about a concept or topic. Mind maps consist of a main topic with branching subtopics and facts coming from the center. More information on mind mapping can be found at http://www.peterrussell.com/MindMaps/HowTo.php.

Morning meeting: A 10–15 minute period in which teachers and students greet one another and do an activity or discuss an issue together. This time helps establish a community and helps both the teacher and students address issues in a safe place rather than having them impact the entire day. (A book on morning meetings is included as a resource in Chapter 12.)

Motivation: A set of reasons for why a person participates in a particular behavior.

Neurotic perfectionism: See Unhealthy perfectionism.

Nonperfectionism: Exhibiting neither the signs of healthy nor unhealthy perfectionism. Underachievers may be mistakenly considered nonperfectionists, although their perfectionistic tendencies might be a reason why they are underachieving.

Normal perfectionism: See Healthy perfectionism.

Observational techniques: Strategies and protocols used in research and educational settings that rely primarily on observations made by teachers or evaluators. These observations may be informal, such as the recording of anecdotes, or formal, such as the use of observation instruments.

Off-peak times: Times when your child is in a calm state, which may be an ideal time to discuss the effects of unhealthy perfectionism.

Other-oriented perfectionism: When a child holds other people to high standards of perfection.

Overextended: A condition that is common among modern children, in which they are overly committed to extracurricular activities.

Parenting style: The way in which parents relate to their children. Parenting styles include authoritarian, authoritative (democratic), and passive.

Peer acceptance: How much a child is accepted by classmates; it is a coping resource that can help children change unhealthy perfectionism to healthy perfectionism.

Perfectionism: A condition in which a person focuses on achieving high goals; it may be healthy or unhealthy.

Perfectionistic behaviors: Behaviors that a person exhibits that are tied to perfectionism, usually interpreted as unhealthy behaviors.

Perfectionistic tendencies: Sometimes also referred to as perfectionistic behaviors, they are the inclination to engage in perfectionism.

Performance goals: Goals that are tied directly to a person's measurable behaviors; goals related to one's own performance, such as improving by a measurable amount.

Personal goals: Goals that are focused on what the child wants to improve, master, and enjoy, rather than on competitive goals like winning a competition or sport.

Pie chart: A graph that divides the whole into proportional parts using a circle. This type of organizer especially is helpful in aiding children to see how to prioritize their time.

Play therapy: Therapy that employs an interpersonal environment to evaluate and modify a child's behavior and cognitions. Popular strategies in play therapy include helping the child identify negative themes within his or her play, providing ways for the child to cope with mistakes and criticism, expanding the child's choices for play materials, helping the child cope with anxiety, and helping the child develop a greater tolerance for mistakes.

Psychological distress: Emotional or behavioral issues that prevent a child or student from normal functioning. Psychological distress sometimes is associated with unhealthy perfectionism.

Preventative measures: Steps taken by parents, teachers, counselors, or other adults to avoid unhealthy outcomes before they happen.

Prioritizing: The process of deciding to give certain tasks and activities more time and attention than other tasks or activities. This can help some types of perfectionists gain a more healthy balance of activities.

Problem-solving strategies: Techniques that teachers and students use to solve problems, either practical and in real-life or as part of the curriculum, such as word problems in mathematics class.

Procrastinating Perfectionist: One type of perfectionist who tends to plan an extensive project but then fails to start it for fear of his or her inability to achieve his or her perfect vision.

Procrastination: Putting off beginning activities or tasks until later, sometimes as a result of perfectionism and a fear of not completing the task to high expectations.

Realistic goal: A goal that can be obtained by a person; it may be based on high expectations but still is manageable given limitations of resources and time.

Risk Evader: A type of perfectionist who has a fear of failure to achieve his or her standards and ideals so he or she chooses not to attempt the task.

Scientific techniques: Strategies used in research settings utilizing measured outcomes, reliable instruments, and the scientific method.

Self-concept: How a person feels about him- or herself; it usually is associated with a domain, such as academic, social, or physical.

Self-criticism: The tendency for some people to critique their own behavior in a negative fashion.

Self-esteem: How a person feels about him- or herself in a global way; it most often is associated with an overall sense of self.

Self-oriented perfectionism: Perfectionism that is characterized by a strong sense of self-motivation. In this type of perfectionism, the child holds him- or herself to extremely high standards.

Short-term goals: Goals that are set for a short period of time, usually between 1 and 3 weeks.

Social confidence: How able a child is able to disclose feelings and opinions in social settings; it is a coping resource that can help children change unhealthy perfectionism to healthy perfectionism.

Socially prescribed perfectionism: A type of perfectionism when children believe that other people hold them to high standards and are critical of their mistakes.

Subtasks: Smaller tasks that are part of a larger goal; by breaking down large tasks into smaller subtasks with concrete deadlines, students may be able to avoid procrastination and may gain a better sense of accomplishment and satisfaction with progress.

Suicide: A serious outcome of psychological distress in which a person takes his or her own life. Unhealthy perfectionism is sometimes associated with a higher risk for suicide.

Summative assessments: Assessments given by teachers, researchers, or other educational professionals at the conclusion of a unit of study. Summative assessments measure the level of mastery of content by students.

Task-involving environments: Home situations in which parents are involved with their children in everyday tasks and family activities.

Teachable moments: Times that parents, teachers, or other adults can use to illustrate a particular lesson or concept. These typically are spontaneous events that occur naturally within the course of the day of which the adult takes advantage to address or teach a particular concept.

Unhealthy perfectionism: Sometimes called *neurotic* or *maladaptive perfectionism*, it is the type of perfectionism that most often comes to mind when parents and teachers think of their children. It represents the perfectionism that causes concern about a student's behavior and well-being and is focused on unrealistic expectations for performance or outcomes. Overly developed self-criticism, stress, procrastination, fear of failure, and risk avoidance are some common signs of unhealthy perfectionism.

Unrealistic goal: A goal that is unattainable given the limitations of resources, time, or ability. Unhealthy perfectionists often hold unrealistic goals for their own performance.

Videotherapy: A type of therapy commonly used with children in which movies are used to address common social or emotional issues.

Well-balanced life: When children have a balance of healthy habits, including proper sleep, exercise, and eating habits, along with academic, extracurricular, social, and recreational time in their lives. This balance may vary from child to child but includes "downtime" along with other objectives.

"WIMI's" ("Why I Missed It"): A strategy used by educators to allow students time for reflection and ensure understanding of concepts covered on an assessment or practice work. (See Figure 15; p. 129.)

REFERENCES

Ablard, K. E., & Parker, W. D. (1997). Parents' achievement goals and perfectionism in their academically talented children. *Journal of Youth and Adolescence, 26,* 651–667.

Adderholdt-Elliott, M. (1987). *Perfectionism: What's bad about being too good.* Minneapolis, MN: Free Spirit.

Adderholdt-Elliot, M. (January/February 1989). Perfectionism and underachievement. *Gifted Child Today,* 19–21.

Adderholdt-Elliott, M., & Eller, S. (1989). Counseling students who are gifted through bibliotherapy. *Teaching Exceptional Children, 22*(1), 26–31.

Adelson, J. L. (2007). A "perfect" case study: Perfectionism in academically talented fourth graders. *Gifted Child Today, 30*(4), 14–20.

Aldea, M. A. (2008). Brief, online interventions for perfectionists. *Dissertation Abstracts International, 68.* (UMI No. 0419-4217)

Amutio, A., & Smith, J. C. (2007). The factor structure of situational and dispositional versions of the Smith Irrational Beliefs Inventory in a Spanish student population. *International Journal of Stress Management, 14,* 321–328.

Arpin-Cribbie, C. A. (2008). Perfectionism related cognitions and psychological distress: A randomized trial evaluating the relative effectiveness of a Web-based cognitive behavioral intervention protocol. *Dissertation Abstracts International, 68.* (UMI No. 0419-4217)

Arpin-Cribbie, C. A., & Cribbie, R. A. (2007). Psychological correlates of fatigue: Examining depression, perfectionism, and automatic negative thoughts. *Personality and Individual Differences, 43,* 1310–1320.

Ashby, J. S., Kottman, T., & Martin, J. L. (2004). Play therapy with young perfectionists. *International Journal of Play Therapy, 13,* 35–55.

Bardone-Cone, A. M. (2007). Self-oriented and socially prescribed perfectionism dimensions and their associations with disordered eating. *Behaviour Research and Therapy, 45,* 1977–1986.

Biran, M. W., & Reese, C. (2007). Parental influences on social anxiety: The sources of perfectionism. *Journal of the American Psychoanalytic Association, 55,* 282–285.

Blankstein, K. R., Dunkley, D. M., & Wilson, J. (2008). Evaluative concerns and personal standards perfectionism: Self-esteem as a mediator and moderator of relations with personal and academic needs and estimated GPA. *Current Psychology, 27,* 29–61.

Blankstein, K. R., Lumley, C. H., & Crawford, A. (2007). Perfectionism, hopelessness, and suicide ideation: Revisions to diathesis-stress and specific vulnerability models. *Journal of Rational-Emotive & Cognitive Behavior Therapy, 25,* 279–319.

Boergers, J., Spirito, A., & Donaldson, D. (1998). Reasons for adolescent suicide attempts: Associations with psychological functioning. *Journal of the American Academy of Child & Adolescent Psychiatry, 37,* 1287–1293.

Böhm, R. (n.d.). *Painting of flowers and birds.* Retrieved January 29, 2009, from http://www.sumi-e-painting.com/sumi-e-galerie-uebersicht-gesamt.htm

Brannan, M. E., & Petrie, T. A. (2008). Moderators of the body dissatisfaction-eating disorder symptomatology relationship: Replication and extension. *Journal of Counseling Psychology, 55,* 263–275.

Calam, R., & Waller, G. (1998). Are eating and psychosocial characteristics in early teenage years useful predictors of eating characteristics in early adulthood? A 7-year longitudinal study. *International Journal of Eating Disorders, 24,* 351–362.

Callard-Szulgit, R. (2003). *Perfectionism and gifted children.* Lanham, MD: Scarecrow Press.

Castro, S., Gula, A., Gual, P., Lahortiga, F., Saura, B. A., & Toro, J. (2004). Perfectionism dimensions in children and adolescents with anorexia nervosa. *Journal of Adolescent Health, 35,* 392–398.

Castro-Fornieles, J., Gual, P., Lahortiga, F., Gila, A., Casulà, V., Fuhrmann, C., et al. (2007). Self-oriented perfectionism in eating disorders. *International Journal of Eating Disorders, 40,* 562–568.

Chan, D. W. (2003). Adjustment problems and multiple intelligences among gifted students in Hong Kong: The development of the revised Student Adjustment Problems Inventory. *High Ability Studies, 14,* 41–54.

Chang, E. C., Ivezaj, V., Downey, C. A., Kashima, Y., & Morady, A. R. (2008). Complexities of measuring perfectionism: Three popular perfectionism measures and their relations with eating disturbances and health behaviors in a female college student sample. *Eating Behaviors, 9,* 102–110.

Chang, E. C., Zumberg, K. M., Sanna, L. J., Girz, L. P., Kade, A. M., Shair, S. R., et al. (2007). Relationship between perfectionism and domains of worry in a college student population: Considering the role of bis/bas motives. *Personality and Individual Differences, 43,* 925–936.

Conners, C. K., Sitarenios, G., Parker, J. D. A., & Epstein, J. N. (1998a). The revised Conners' Parent Rating Scale (CPRS-R): Factor structure, reliability, and criterion validity. *Journal of Abnormal Child Psychology, 26,* 257–268.

Conners, C. K., Sitarenios, G., Parker, J. D. A., & Epstein, J. N. (1998b). Revision and restandardization of the Conners' Teacher Rating Scale (CTRS-R): Factor structure, reliability, and criterion validity. *Journal of Abnormal Child Psychology, 26,* 279–291.

Daigneault, S. D. (1999). Narrative means to Adlerian ends: An illustrated comparison of narrative therapy and Adlerian play therapy. *Journal of Individual Psychology, 55,* 298–315.

Dekryger, N. A. (2006). Childhood perfectionism: Measurement, phenomenology, and development. *Dissertation Abstracts International, 67.* (UMI No. 0419-4217)

Diprima, A. J. (2003). The relationship between family variables and perfectionism in middle school students. *Dissertation Abstracts International, 64.* (UMI No. 0419-4209)

Dixon, F. A., Lapsley, D. K., & Hanchon, T. A. (2004). An empirical typology of perfectionism in gifted adolescents. *Gifted Child Quarterly, 48,* 95–106.

Downey, C. A., & Chang, E. C. (2007). Perfectionism and symptoms of eating disturbances in female college students: Considering the role of negative affect and body dissatisfaction. *Eating Behaviors, 8,* 497–503.

Egan, S. J., Piek, J. P., Dyck, M. J., & Rees, C. S. (2007). The role of dichotomous thinking and rigidity in perfectionism. *Behaviour Research and Therapy, 45,* 1813–1822.

Flamenbaum, R., & Holden, R. R. (2007). Psychache as a mediator in the relationship between perfectionism and suicidality. *Journal of Counseling Psychology, 54,* 51–61.

Frasier, M. M., & McCannon, C. (1981). Using bibliotherapy with gifted children. *Gifted Child Quarterly, 25,* 81–85.

Flett, G. L., Hewitt, P. L., Blankenstein, K. R., & Pickering, D. (1998). Perfectionism in relation to attributions for success or failure. *Current Psychology, 17,* 249–262.

Flett, G. L., Hewitt, P. L., Whelan, T., & Martin, T. R. (2007). The Perfectionism Cognitions Inventory: Psychometric properties and associations with distress and deficits in cognitive self-management. *Journal of Rational-Emotive & Cognitive Behavior Therapy, 25,* 255–277.

Frost, R. O., Lahart, C. M., & Rosnblate, R. (1991). The development of perfectionism: A study of daughters and their parents. *Cognitive Therapy and Research, 15,* 469–489.

Frost, R. O., & Marten, P. A. (1990). Perfectionism and evaluative threat. *Cognitive Therapy and Research, 14,* 559–572.

Gallucci, N. T., Middleton, G., & Kline, A. (2000). Perfectionism and creative strivings. *Journal of Creative Behavior, 34,* 135–141.

Gaspar, S. (2007). Children of Alcoholics in Recovery and Educational program (CARE): Education and treatment for children of alcoholic parents. *Dissertation Abstracts International, 68.* (UMI No. 0419-4217)

Gilman, R., & Ashby, J. S. (2003). Multidimensional perfectionism in a sample of middle school students: An exploratory investigation. *Psychology in the Schools, 40,* 677–689.

Greenspon, T. S. (2008). Making sense of error: A view of the origins and treatment of perfectionism. *American Journal of Psychotherapy, 62,* 263–282.

Hamachek, D. E. (1978). Psychodynamics of normal and neurotic perfectionism. *Psychology: A Journal of Human Behavior, 15,* 27–33.

Hawkins, C. C., Watt, H. M. G., & Sinclair, K. E. (2006). Psychometric properties of the Frost Multidimensional Perfectionism Scale with Australian adolescent girls: Clarification of multidimensionality and perfectionist typology. *Educational and Psychological Measurement, 66,* 1001–1022.

Hébert, T. (1991, June). Meeting the affective needs of bright boys through bibliotherapy. *Roeper Review, 13,* 207–212.

Hébert, T. (2009). Guiding gifted teenagers to self-understanding through biography. In J. L. VanTassel-Baska, T. L. Cross, & F. R. Olenchak (Eds.), *Social-*

emotional curriculum with gifted and talented students (pp. 259–288). Waco, TX: Prufrock Press.

Hewitt, P. L., Caelian, C. F., Flett, G. L., Sherry, S. B., Collins, L., & Flynn, C. A. (2002). Perfectionism in children: Associations with depression, anxiety, and anger. *Personality and Individual Differences, 32,* 1049–1061.

Hewitt, P. L., Newton, J., Flett, G. L., & Callander, L. (1997). Perfectionism and suicide ideation in adolescent psychiatric patients. *Journal of Abnormal Child Psychology, 25,* 95–101.

Huprich, S. K., Porcerelli, J., Keaschuk, R., Binienda, J., & Engle, B. (2008). Depressive personality disorder, dysthymia, and their relationship to perfectionism. *Depression and Anxiety, 25,* 207–217.

Immundsen, Y., Roberts, G. C., Lemyre, P.-N., & Miller, B. W. (2005). Peer relationships in adolescent competitive soccer: Associations to perceived motivational climate, achievement goals and perfectionism. *Journal of Sports Sciences, 23,* 977–989.

Internet Public Library. (2007). *Avi.* Retrieved from http://www.ipl.org/div/askauthor/Avi.html

Jones, S. A. (2008). An experimental analysis of the relationship between perfectionism and depressive mood. *Dissertation Abstracts International, 68.* (UMI No. 0419-4217)

Kearns, H., Forbes, A., & Gardiner, M. (2007). A cognitive behavioural coaching intervention for the treatment of perfectionism and self-handicapping in a nonclinical population. *Behaviour Change, 24,* 157–172.

Kearns, H., Gardiner, M., & Marshall, K. (2008). Innovation in Ph.D. completion: The hardy shall succeed (and be happy!). *Higher Education Research & Development, 27,* 77–89.

Kenney-Benson, G. A., & Pomerantz, E. M. (2005). The role of mothers' use of control in children's perfectionism: Implications for the development of children's depressive symptoms. *Journal of Personality, 73,* 23–46.

Kline, B. E., & Short, E. B. (1991). Changes in emotional resilience: Gifted adolescent females. *Roeper Review, 13,* 118–121.

Kowal, A., & Pritchard, D. W. (1990). Psychological characteristics of children who suffer from headache: A research note. *Journal of Child Psychology and Psychiatry, 31,* 637–649.

Laurenti, H. J., Bruch, M. A., & Haase, R. F. (2008). Social anxiety and socially prescribed perfectionism: Unique and interactive relationships with maladaptive appraisal of interpersonal situations. *Personality and Individual Differences, 45*, 55–61.

Leon, G. R., Kendall, P. C., & Garber, J. (1980). Depression in children: Parent, teacher, and child perspectives. *Journal of Abnormal Child Psychology, 8*, 221–235.

LoCicero, K. A., & Ashby, J. S. (2000). Multidimensional perfectionism in middle school age gifted students: A comparison to peers from the general cohort. *Roeper Review, 22*, 182–185.

March, J. S., Parker, J. D. A., Sullivan, K., & Stallings, P. (1997). The Multidimensional Anxiety Scale for Children (MASC): Factor structure, reliability, and validity. *Journal of the American Academy of Child & Adolescent Psychiatry, 36*, 554–565.

McArdle, S., & Duda, J. L. (2004). Exploring social-contextual correlates of perfectionism in adolescents: A multivariate perspective. *Cognitive Therapy and Research, 28*, 765–788.

McCreary, B. T., Joiner, T. E., Schmidt, N. B., & Ialongo, N. S. (2004). The structure and correlates of perfectionism in African American children. *Journal of Clinical Child and Adolescent Psychology, 33*, 313–324.

Morelock, M. J. (1992). Giftedness: The view from within. *Understanding Our Gifted, 4*(3), 1, 11–15.

Must, S. (2008). The dual effects of parenting and perfectionism on maladjustment and academic performance of affluent suburban adolescents. *Dissertation Abstracts International, 68*. (UMI No. 0419-4217)

Nounopoulos, A., Ashby, J. S., & Gilman, R. (2006). Coping resources, perfectionism, and academic performance among adolescents. *Psychology in the Schools, 43*, 613–622.

O'Brien, D. R. (2006). Distinguishing between students with and without learning disabilities: A comparative analysis of cognition, achievement, perceptual skills, behavior, and executive functioning. *Dissertation Abstracts International, 67* (3-A). (UMI No. AA13209081)

O'Connor, R. C. (2007). The relations between perfectionism and suicidality: A systematic review. *Suicide and Life-Threatening Behavior, 37*, 698–714.

O'Leary, N., & Schuler, P. A. (2003, November). *Perfectionism in parents of gifted students*. Paper presented at the annual conference of the National Association for Gifted Children, Indianapolis, IN.

Parker, W. D. (1997). An empirical typology of perfectionism in academically talented children. *American Educational Research Journal, 34,* 545–562.

Parker, W. D. (2000). Healthy perfectionism in the gifted. *Journal of Secondary Gifted Education, 11,* 173–182.

Parker, W. D., Flett, G. L., & Hewitt, P. L. (2002). Perfectionism and adjustment in gifted children. In G. L. Flett & P. L. Hewitt (Eds.), *Perfectionism: Theory, research, and treatment* (pp. 133–148). Washington, DC: American Psychological Association.

Parker, W. D., Portesova, S., & Stumpf, H. (2001). Perfectionism in mathematically gifted and typical Czech students. *Journal for the Education of the Gifted, 25,* 138–152.

Parker, W. D., & Mills, C. J. (1996). The incidence of perfectionism in gifted students. *Gifted Child Quarterly, 40,* 194–199.

Parker, W. D., & Stumpf, H. (1995). An examination of the Multidimensional Perfectionism Scale with a sample of academically talented children. *Journal of Psychoeducational Assessment, 13,* 372–383.

Pritchard, M. E., Wilson, G. S., & Yamnitz, B. (2007). What predicts adjustment among college students? A longitudinal panel study. *Journal of American College Health, 56,* 15–21.

Renzulli, J. S. (1986). The three-ring conception of giftedness: A developmental model for creative productivity. In R. J. Sternberg & J. Davidson (Eds.), *Conceptions of giftedness* (pp. 53–92). New York: Cambridge University Press.

Rice, K. G., Ashby, J. S., & Slaney, R. B. (2007). Perfectionism and the five-factor model of personality. *Assessment, 14,* 385–398.

Rice, K. G., & Dellwo, J. P. (2002). Perfectionism and self-development: Implications for college adjustment. *Journal of Counseling and Development, 80,* 188–196.

Rice, K. G., Kubal, A. E., & Preusser, K. J. (2004). Perfectionism and children's self-concept: Further validation of the adaptive/maladaptive perfectionism scale. *Psychology in the Schools, 41,* 279–290.

Rice, K. G., Leever, B. A., Noggle, C. A., & Lapsley, D. K. (2007). Perfectionism and depressive symptoms in early adolescence. *Psychology in the Schools, 44,* 139–156.

Riley, C., Lee, M., Cooper, Z., Fairburn, C. G., & Shafran, R. (2007). A randomised controlled trial of cognitive-behaviour therapy for clinical perfectionism: A preliminary study. *Behaviour Research and Therapy, 45,* 2221–2231.

Saddler, C. D., & Buckland, R. L. (1995). The Multidimensional Perfectionism Scale: Correlations with depression in college students with learning disabilities. *Psychological Reports, 77,* 483–490.

Schuler, P. A. (2000). Perfectionism and the gifted adolescent. *Journal of Secondary Gifted Education, 11,* 183–196.

Schuler, P. A., Ferbezer, L., O'Leary, N., Popova, L., Delou, C. M. C., & Limont, W. (2003). Perfectionism: International case studies. *Gifted and Talented International, 18,* 67–75.

Siegle, D., & Schuler, P. A. (2000). Perfectionism differences in gifted middle school students. *Roeper Review, 23,* 39–44.

Silverman, L. K. (1993a). A developmental model for counseling the gifted. In L. K. Silverman (Ed.), *Counseling the gifted and talented* (pp. 51–78). Denver, CO: Love.

Silverman, L. K. (1993b). The gifted individual. In L. K. Silverman (Ed.), *Counseling the gifted and talented* (pp. 3–28). Denver, CO: Love

Smith, J. C., Rausch, S. M., & Jenks, J. D. (2004). Factor structure of the Smith Irrational Beliefs Inventory: Results of analyses on six independent samples. *Psychological Reports, 95,* 696–704.

Sondergeld, T. A., Schultz, R. A., & Glover, L. K. (2007). The need for research replication: An example from studies on perfectionism and early gifted adolescents. *Roeper Review, 29*(5), 19–25.

Speirs Neumeister, K. L. (2004). Understanding the relationship between perfectionism and achievement motivation in gifted college students. *Gifted Child Quarterly, 48,* 219–231.

Stoeber, J., Harris, R. A., & Moon, P. S. (2007). Perfectionism and the experience of pride, shame, and guilt: Comparing healthy perfectionists, unhealthy perfectionists, and non-perfectionists. *Personality and Individual Differences, 43,* 131–141.

Stoltz, K., & Ashby, J. S. (2007). Perfectionism and lifestyle: Personality differences among adaptive perfectionists, maladaptive perfectionists, and nonperfectionists. *Journal of Individual Psychology, 63,* 414–423.

Stumpf, H., & Parker, W. D. (2000). A hierarchical structural analysis of perfectionism and its relation to other personality characteristics. *Personality and Individual Differences, 28,* 837–852.

Suddarth, B. H., & Slaney, R. B. (2001). An investigation of the dimensions of perfectionism in college students. *Measurement and Evaluation in Counseling and Development, 34,* 157–165.

Tannenbaum, A. J. (1992). Early signs of giftedness: Research and commentary. *Journal for the Education of the Gifted, 13,* 22–36.

Vallance, J. K. H., Dunn, J. G. H., & Dunn, J. L. C. (2006). Perfectionism, anger, and situation criticality in competitive youth ice hockey. *Journal of Sport & Exercise Psychology, 28,* 383–406.

Vandiver, B. J., & Worrell, F. C. (2002). The reliability and validity of scores on the Almost Perfect Scale—Revised with academically talented middle school students. *Journal of Secondary Gifted Education, 13,* 108–119.

Waller, G., Wood, A., Miller, J., & Slade, P. (1992). The development of neurotic perfectionism: A risk factor for unhealthy eating attitudes. *British Review of Bulimia & Anorexia Nervosa, 6*(2), 57–62.

Wilson, H. E., & Adelson, J. L. (2008, Winter). Art across the curriculum: Language arts. *Teaching for High Potential, 3.*

Witcher, L. A., Alexander, E. S., Onwuebuzie, A. J., Collins, K. M. T., & Witcher, A. E. (2007). The relationship between psychology students' levels of perfectionism and achievement in a graduate-level research methodology course. *Personality and Individual Differences, 43,* 1396–1405.

ABOUT THE AUTHORS

Jill L. Adelson, Ph.D., has worked with children in a variety of settings, including academic, extracurricular, and athletics. She taught fourth-grade self-contained gifted and talented in Newport News, VA, and some of her coaching activities included Odyssey of the Mind, softball, and the academic team. While teaching, Jill earned her master's degree in curriculum and instruction, specializing in gifted education, from The College of William and Mary. As a teacher and graduate student, she conducted case studies on perfectionism in her own classroom. Jill left Virginia to pursue her doctorate in educational psychology with a joint specialization in gifted education and in measurement, evaluation, and assessment at the University of Connecticut, where she worked with students through Project M³: Mentoring Mathematical Minds and Project M²: Mentoring Young Mathematicians. Currently, Jill is an assistant professor at the University of Louisville in educational and counseling psychology. When not conducting research and teaching, she enjoys spending time with her husband, kickboxing, riding her Harley Davidson, and running. A perfectionist herself, Jill understands the benefits of healthy perfectionism as well as the stress and struggles of unhealthy perfectionism.

Hope E. Wilson, Ph.D., writes this book from both the perspective of a parent and an educator. As an educator, she has worked primarily as an elementary art teacher in Texas. In this position, she had the joy of teaching all of the students, from kindergarten through fifth grade, and working with the other teachers to develop cross-curricular activities and connections. Hope earned her master's degree in teaching from Austin College in Sherman, TX, and then a second master's degree in gifted education from Hardin-Simmons University in Abilene, TX. After 4 years of teaching, Hope went to the University of Connecticut to pursue her Ph.D. in educational psychology with a specialization in gifted education. While at the University of Connecticut, Hope was the assistant editor for the *Journal of Advanced Academics* and worked on a variety of research projects. She is the mother of two children, Lily and Keenan. Along with her children and her husband, Jon, she lives in Texas. A life-long perfectionist herself, having children made Hope really consider priorities and refocus her life in order to change unhealthy perfectionism into the more healthy variety.